THE AVAILABILITY OF CARE

for Late-Middle-Aged Adults With Chronic Conditions

THE AVAILABILITY OF CARE

for Late-Middle-Aged Adults With Chronic Conditions

Julie C. Lima and Susan M. Allen

CAMBRIA
PRESS

Amherst, New York

Requests for permission should be directed to:
permissions@cambriapress.com, or mailed to:
Cambria Press
20 Northpointe Parkway, Suite 188
Amherst, NY 14228

Library of Congress Cataloging-in-Publication Data

Lima, Julie C.
The availability of care for late-middle-aged adults with chronic conditions / by Julie C. Lima, Susan M. Allen.
p. cm.
Includes bibliographical references and index.
ISBN 978-1-60497-576-5 (alk. paper)
1. Middle aged persons—Care. 2. Caregivers. 3. Communities. I. Allen, Susan, 1949– II. Title.

HQ1059.4.L54 2008
362.16—dc22

2008047938

To our families, with love

Table of Contents

List of Figures

List of Tables

Preface

When asked, each of us could probably name one or more family members and/or friends who are providing care in the community to ailing parents or elderly spouses. Given a bit more time, I bet that we could also think of someone who is not yet of retirement age, but who also needs assistance with everyday activities due to an acute or chronic condition. Just within my immediate circle of family I can think of three relatives who required care before the age of 65. My godfather was diagnosed with multiple sclerosis (MS) in his 40s and declined for 20 years before succumbing to the disease in December 2004. Another uncle was given months to live after being diagnosed with brain cancer in his 50s, but lived an additional 4 years. Finally, my mother-in-law has been fighting the effects of hereditary heart disease and other ailments since her late 30s, but now, at 60, is feeling the effects that more than a decade of antirejection medication can have on the body.

All three scenarios are so very different and yet the everyday reality was strikingly similar. All three relatives required around-the-clock care over an extended period of time. All three had spouses who assumed the bulk of that care and who changed their work schedules or left their jobs altogether. They also have sons and daughters who helped out, and whose own lives and careers have been significantly impacted by their caregiving responsibilities. But, in a sense, all three families were better situated than the average American to handle their situations. Both of my uncles and my mother-in-law had spouses who were willing and able to take on the primary caregiver role. Two had either a spouse or child who was a nurse by profession. All were fortunate enough to have a least one pension to rely on when it became too difficult to manage both caregiving and work.

Despite the many resources available to my relatives, caregiving was a daily struggle, causing me to wonder how other Americans in similar circumstances fare. Divorce rates are high, pensions are quickly becoming a thing of the past, and most family caregivers do not have formal training in a health care profession. As I am writing this preface, Congress has just voted a $700 billion "bailout" of financial institutions in an effort to bolster our failing economy, and unemployment rates are higher than they have been in years, with predictions of more job loss to come. Medicaid programs are searching for ways to cut costs in the face of increasing need. Balancing work and family obligations in this economic climate will be a daunting challenge.

This study was the first to focus attention on the care needs of individuals who needed assistance "prematurely." Prematurely, however, is a misnomer, as more than 1.4 million Americans aged 55–64 had limitations in physical or cognitive functioning at the time of this study. We highlight availability and amount of care for this group compared to their counterparts at older ages who are eligible to benefit from the safety net of Medicare and social security retirement income, and who are more likely to have a spouse who is retired and able to provide care without competing employment obligations. What we found was not always encouraging, but will hopefully lead to more research into the needs of this overlooked group.

Acknowledgments

This study was funded in part by a Demography Fellowship from the National Institute for Child Health and Human Development. Portions of these analyses are also reported in Lima, Allen, Goldscheider, and Intrator (2008)'s article, "Spousal Caregiving in Late Midlife Versus Older Ages: Implications of work and Family Obligations," in *Journal of Gerontology: Social Sciences*. The Health and Retirement Study (HRS) is sponsored by the National Institute on Aging (grant number NIA U01AG009740) and is conducted by the University of Michigan. We would like to thank Frances Goldscheider and Orna Intrator for their guidance early on in the process. Dr. Goldscheider provided guidance with the conceptualization of the study, and Dr. Intrator advised the statistical analyses, suggesting imputation techniques and sensitivity analyses to strengthen the methods and confirm the results. We would also like to thank Cambria Press for their interest in our work and their flexibility and guidance throughout the entire process.

List of Abbreviations

ADL	activities of daily living
AHEAD	Assets and Health Dynamics of the Oldest Old
AoA	Administration on Aging
BMI	body mass index
CDC	Centers for Disease Control and Prevention
CMS	Centers for Medicare and Medicaid Services
HRS	Health and Retirement Study
IADL	instrumental activities of daily living
ICF	International Classification of Functioning, Disability and Health (formerly ICIDH)
NHIS-D	National Health Interview Survey on Disability
NIA	National Institute on Aging
TICS	Telephone Interview for Cognitive Status
WHO	World Health Organization

THE AVAILABILITY OF CARE

for Late-Middle-Aged Adults With Chronic Conditions

Chapter 1

Introduction

Among the most critical issues facing society today is the provision of community support for people of all ages who require assistance to perform daily living tasks. Researchers have documented the support systems and needs of older persons, children with special health care needs, and young persons transitioning into adulthood. While the United States may not yet have solved many of the challenges of providing adequate supports to these populations, researchers at least have a good sense of the nature of those challenges and are working toward that end. Somewhat surprising, then, is their nearly complete lack of knowledge about the support systems and needs of a rapidly growing population of adults who are not yet considered old but who nevertheless need help due to traumatic injury, the congenital illnesses of childhood and young adulthood, and/or the early onset of chronic diseases typically associated with later life, for example, arthritis, heart disease, and cancer. Specifically, researchers know little about the millions of Americans who require assistance during the period of late middle age, a transition phase between middle age and the older years, when activity limitations associated with a chronic condition escalate sharply, with an estimated 12% of people aged 45–54 and 20% of people aged 55–64 reporting such limitations (Pastor, Makuc, Reuben, & Xia, 2002).

By assistance with daily living tasks, we mean help with activities of daily living (ADLs), such as walking, bathing, dressing, eating, toileting, and transferring into and out of bed. We also mean help with instrumental activities of daily living (IADLs), such as grocery shopping, managing money, using the telephone, doing housework, getting around outside, cooking, and managing medications. Taken for granted by most, it is easy to understand how an unmet need for assistance with these activities would make it very difficult, and for some impossible, to live in the community. Indeed, unmet need for ADLs and IADLs has been linked to such negative consequences as burns, falls, and even institutionalization (Gaugler, Kane, Kane, & Newcomer, 2005; LaPlante, Kaye, Kang, & Harrington, 2004).

OBJECTIVES OF THE STUDY

This study fills a critical gap in the literature to date. Using a nationally representative sample, we are the first to focus attention on the self-care needs of this age group. We examined the characteristics of persons in late middle age with limitations in function. We took a close look at their potential support systems and at the amount of care that they received, and we explored reasons why they may or may not have gotten adequate care from their support networks. Throughout the study, we compared their characteristics, their care networks, and the amount of care they received to those of people in older age groups. In this book, we discuss current and planned strategies to assist older persons and considered whether they might also benefit this younger group, or whether we need to consider entirely new initiatives. Finally, we lay the groundwork for future research in this area.

Significance

Can there really be that many people who are sick enough to require assistance before age 65? The answer is yes. In 2002 an estimated 5% of this age group, approximately 1.4 million Americans, reported needing assistance with daily activities as a result of a severe disability (Steinmetz, 2006). Recent studies suggest that morbid obesity and resultant chronic conditions are on the rise among people over 50, as well as younger age groups (McTigue et al., 2006; O'Rand, 2005). Trends in obesity coupled with the aging of the 78 million–strong baby boom generation—the oldest of whom turned 60 in 2006—ensure that these numbers will only increase in the near future.

At first glance, people in late middle age appear to be ideally situated if a need arises—they have both older and younger generations to call upon for assistance, and they are more likely than other age groups to be married (U.S. Census Bureau, 2007). Availability of assistance, however, does not automatically translate into assistance received. In fact, there are reasons to expect that there are fewer helping resources available to people in late middle age who are "prematurely" in need of help. First, family and friends may have time constraints. For example, people who are disabled before age 65 may receive less help from their children than older groups given that their children may still be dependent, or may be starting families and careers during the early stages of adult life when time demands are high. Spousal assistance may be weighed against a depletion in savings and potentially a loss of health insurance coverage if the spouse must leave the workforce to provide assistance, scenarios less likely for an older couple who is likely already retired and covered by Medicare. Indeed, people in late middle age in general are at high risk for being uninsured as they transition out of work but are too young for universal coverage under Medicare (Pol, Mueller, & Adidam, 2000).

Cohort differences may exacerbate problems in access to helping resources for late-middle-aged adults with disabilities at the turn of the 21st century. They are the baby boomers and pre-boomers, characterized by a higher rate of divorce and a lower rate of remarriage, a lower rate of fertility and later child bearing, and a higher proportion of women with extensive work histories than today's older cohorts. Thus, on the one hand, both life stage and social cohort effects may compound the problem of family availability to provide help to people with functional limitation in late middle age. On the other hand, the increased labor force participation of women may potentially allow for more paid assistance. How these life course issues actually play out in terms of differences in care arrangements has not been studied.

Clearly, work in this area was long overdue. The merging of the Health and Retirement Study (HRS) and the Assets and Health Dynamics of the Oldest Old (AHEAD) data sets, the premier sources of information on resources, health, and well-being, made it possible to examine these questions. We made use of the 2000 survey, a representative sample of noninstitutionalized adults aged 50 and older in the United States.

The final two sections of this chapter provide a road map for the rest of the book. We first provide definitions that are critical to the understanding of the entire discussion. We end this chapter by outlining the chapters that follow.

Key Definitions

Age Groups: Late Middle Age, Young Old, and Older Old

Generally, older persons (formally referred to in the literature as *elderly*) are considered to be ages 65 and older. In this study, three age groups were distinguished. We differentiated between people who were "young old" and "older old," given that today, people aged 65–74 are considered to be a transitional group, eligible for Medicare, aging services, and social security benefits, yet are still more likely to be working and have other dependents than those who are older old. Therefore, we referred to those aged 50–64 as people in late middle age, those 65–74 as people who were young old, and those 75 and older as people who were older old. Any reference to elders more generally refers to those 65 and older.

Life Course, Life Stage, and Cohort

The life course perspective (Elder, 1994) framed the concepts surrounding the receipt of care at late midlife versus old age. Throughout this study, we used *life course* as an umbrella term that encompassed four central themes: "the interplay of human lives and historical times, the timing of lives, linked or interdependent lives, and human agency in choice making" (Elder, p. 5). Both life stage and cohort, to follow, were encompassed within this term. We used *life stage* to refer to aspects associated with the developmental timing of an individual's life. For example, at this point in their life stage, those in late middle age are less likely than those who are older old to have adult children and more likely to have living parents. Finally, *cohort* is generally used to describe a group of individuals who have something in common. For example, one could define a cohort in terms of academic achievement, and so anyone who had a college degree would be a member of one cohort while anyone with at most a high school diploma would be a member of a different cohort. We defined cohorts by age, that is, individuals born within the same span of years were considered to share a cohort. This concept refers best to what Elder described as "the interplay of human lives and historical times." As he noted, for example, the historical impact of World War II was much different for individuals who had already entered adulthood in the 1940s compared with those who were infants at the time. Similarly, the demographic and family transitions that have occurred in the United States since then affected these two groups differently, as we discuss in chapter 2.

Functional Limitation

Any study involving the receipt of community-based care must begin with a definition of those who may need or receive this care. We focused on individuals who stated that they have difficulty performing one or more ADLs or IADLs, defined previously.

Referring to individuals in this study as having a functional limitation rather than a disability was intentional, particularly in light of the revised paradigm of functioning, disability, and health put forward by the World Health Organization (WHO) in 2001 in the International Classification of Functioning, Disability and Health (referred to here as ICF, and previously also as ICIDH). The ICF framework considers individual, social, and environmental factors in its conceptual framework of disability and health (World Health Organization [WHO], 2001). Its most recent iteration focuses on disability as a continuum that is present in everyone's life, rather than as a state into which an individual either falls or does not. It combines both a medical and social model that focuses not only on individual behaviors and health maintenance but also on social and environmental

FIGURE 1.1. World Health Organization ICF classification.

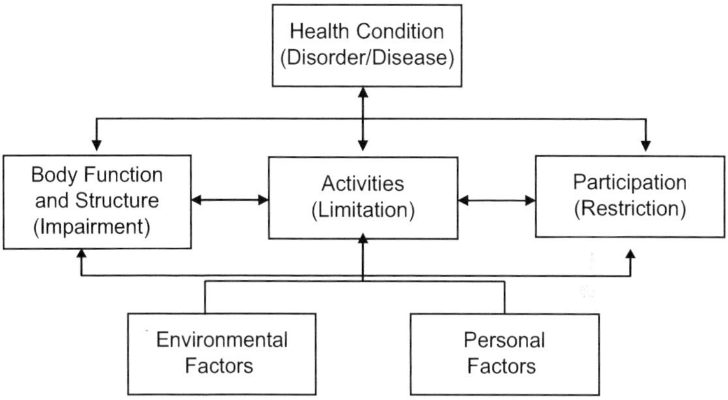

Source. WHO (2001).

factors that enable or hinder the desired end point of participation (WHO, 2001). This model was ideal for the study of the middle-aged population because it did not equate functional limitation with dependence. Figure 1.1 displays graphically the interactive nature of the classification system.

Casemix

We used the term *casemix* to denote a group of indicators that describe the respondents' overall health and functional status. Casemix was inclusive of the number of ADL and IADL difficulties, general health rating, number of nights spent in a hospital over the previous 2 years, number of days spent at home in bed over the previous month, cognitive impairment, pain, number of medical conditions, psychological disorder, exhaustion, use of a wheelchair, and body mass index (BMI).

Noticeably missing from this group was the presence of specific medical conditions, aside from psychological disorders.

Most of the conditions asked about in the HRS are naturally correlated with age, but in themselves say nothing about one's functional/health status so important to needing assistance that is not already captured in the other variables previously mentioned. If a medical condition results in need for assistance, it is through the bodily limitations it imposes. In fact, controlling for them would potentially mask a possible age effect. The presence of a psychological disorder is different from other conditions, however, in that it has historically been stigmatizing to be labeled with a psychological disorder—and this stigma may affect the availability of care. Because psychological disorders were more prevalent among younger cohorts, we controlled for them in all analyses.

Community-Based Care

Here, community-based care referred to any combination of the use of community-based services, including informal (unpaid) help from family and friends, as well as formal (paid) help. Institutionalization, rare among people in late middle age, was not considered in this study. Institutionalization refers specifically to living in a nursing home. The Health and Retirement Study (2000) provided the following definition of nursing home in its survey instrument: "A nursing home provides all of the following services for its residents: dispensing of medications, 24-hour nursing assistance and supervision, personal assistance, and room and meals" (p. 6, Coverscreen questionnaire). Respondents who lived in retirement or assisted living communities were considered to be living in the community; therefore, care provided by these residences was considered community-based care. We used other terms throughout the study to denote various aspects of community-based care, such as supports, formal and/or informal care/help, helping networks, and care networks.

Support/Care Network, Social Network

The distinction between these two terms is particularly important in understanding the theoretical framework. Drawing from Faber and Wasserman (2001), the support network (sometimes referred to as the care network) referred to the individuals who actually provided hands-on assistance to persons with functional limitations. The social network, however, referred to people who were tied together through relationships and who may share resources. In this study, these were immediate family or household members who were present in the respondent's life, but who may or may not have provided hands-on help. We considered these people to be potential helpers.

Format of the Remaining Chapters

The focus of this study was on age differences in the receipt and amount of care provided to persons 50 and older living in the community with functional limitations. In chapter 2, we present the theoretical framework used to inform our hypotheses, expand the discussion surrounding the importance of this study in space and time (i.e., the United States in 2000), and provide a brief summary of caregiving research to date before presenting our formal hypotheses. In chapter 3, we describe the data and methods used to achieve our goals.

Chapter 4 is the first analytic chapter. In it, we examine age differences in the receipt of care among individuals with an ADL/IADL difficulty. In chapter 5, and all remaining analytic chapters, we narrow the sample to those individuals with ADL/IADL difficulties who received at least a minimum amount of care, and examine age differences in the structure of the care network. In chapter 6, we examine age differences in the amount of care (measured in hours) received by sample members, with a particular focus on the amount of care provided by the primary caregiver. In chapter 7, we examine the characteristics of two specific types of primary caregivers—spouses and children—and determine how these characteristics affect the amount of care that they provided. Finally, in chapter 8, we summarize the findings and outline policy implications. Using our findings as a springboard, we also outline a research agenda that will further advance our understanding of the needs of people in late middle age.

Chapter 2

Background, Theory, and Hypotheses

Theoretical Framework

The task-specificity model of caregiving (Litwak, 1985) embedded within the life course perspective (also referred to as a *theoretical orientation*, *framework*, or *paradigm* in the literature—see Ajrouch, Antonucci, & Janevic, 2001; Elder & Johnson, 2002; George, 2002; Settersten, 2002) informed the specific hypotheses in this study. Elder (1994) attributed the emergence of the life course perspective to the integration of "various theoretical strands including the macro world of age stratification (Elder, 1975; Riley, Johnson, and Foner 1972), cultural and intergenerational models (Kertzer and Keith 1984), and developmental life span psychology (Baltes 1987)" (p. 5). A relatively new perspective, since the 1990s it has had a major role in the framing of studies surrounding families in the middle and later years (Allen, Blieszner, & Roberto, 2000). It emphasizes the importance of considering human lives and choices in the context of the broader social structure and historical time, as well as the developmental timing of lives within these broader social structures. Put another way, a person's life course consists of a series of transitions and trajectories that are taking place within a specific historical context and personal biography, and are affected by the interdependence of the individual's life with the lives of others (George, 2002). Individuals and their circumstances, therefore, cannot be studied in isolation.

Just as the timing of a health transition (i.e., the age at which a person becomes ill) may have important consequences for the course of the illness (George, 2002), the timing may also have important consequences on the type and amount of help a person receives when their functioning becomes limited. Individuals who require assistance with activities of daily living rely, for the most part, on the support of other individuals. As the life course perspective suggests, the amount and type of this support depends not only on the characteristics of the individual in need (e.g., demographics, functional capacity, resources, and preferences) but also on the characteristics of his or her available social network and support. These characteristics reflect both the developmental stage of the life condition (i.e., being functionally limited in late midlife vs. old age) and historical timing of individual lives (i.e., the demographic and family transitions of the late 20th century have differentially affected today's late-middle-aged, young old, and older old cohorts). Both of these two concepts are examined further in later text.

Litwak's task-specificity model as applied to caregiving suggests that there is an order that is followed when choosing caregivers

(Litwak, 1985; Messeri, Silverstein, & Litwak, 1993). Litwak demonstrated that optimal informal support groups were chosen based on four dimensions: proximity, length of commitment, commonality of lifestyle or major social roles, and size. In the case of caregiving, spouses and children are generally the closest in proximity and have the greatest commitment level compared with other groups. This proximity and the commitment level are important, given that a need for care may arise at any point during the day or night (Litwak). In addition, ADL and IADL tasks themselves do not require that an individual have a common lifestyle with the person in need in order to carry out the task. Children, as well as same-aged adults (e.g., spouses), can successfully assume the role. Nor do the caregiving tasks require any special knowledge on the part of the caregiver, eliminating the necessity for a formally trained individual. And because the majority of care provided to individuals in need comes from the primary caregiver, in the case of caregiving, the size of the social network should not be as important as the composition of the network (Messeri et al., 1993).

Litwak's model predicted, and research on the elder population confirmed, that spouses and children are indeed the most prevalent caregivers to older persons, followed by other relatives, friends, and finally nonrelatives (Jette, Tennstedt, & Branch, 1992; Kemper, 1988; Stone, Cafferata, & Sangl, 1987, Wolff & Kasper, 2006). But though Litwak's task-specificity model suggests that the optimal choice of caregivers will follow a similar order for all age groups, the life course perspective hints at potential age differences in the amount of care available to these individuals. Many factors influence the structure of one's social network and the amount of support provided by this network, including the characteristics of the individual and those of their

FIGURE 2.1. Theoretical framework.

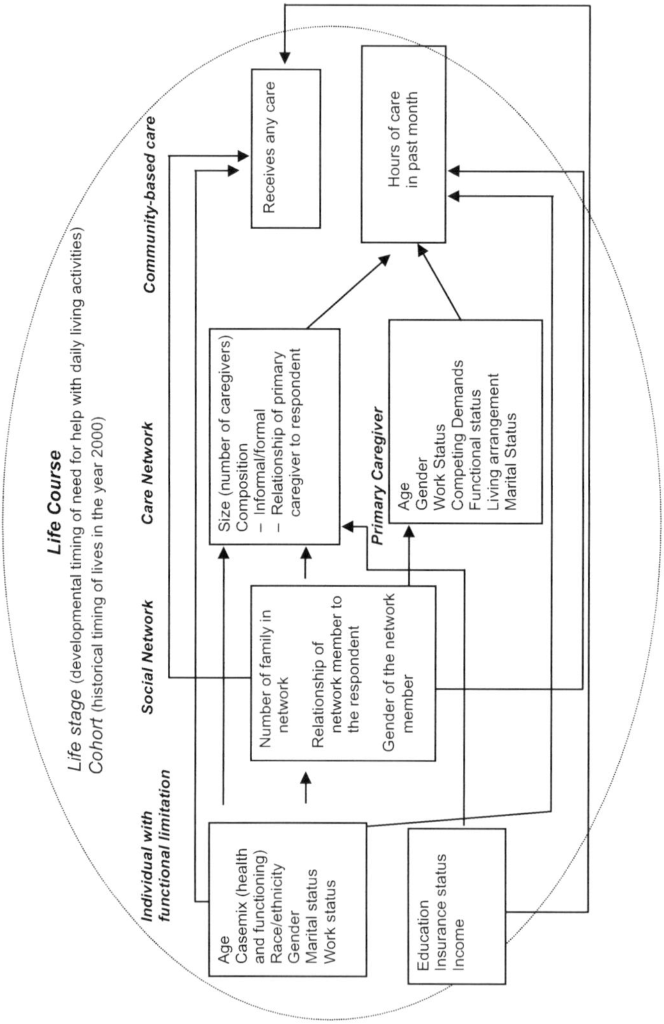

network members (Faber & Wasserman, 2001). Furthermore, the characteristics of the social network as a whole, such as total network size, density, and role structure, contribute to the amount and type of support an individual receives (Faber & Wasserman).

Figure 2.1 depicts the interplay of the characteristics of care receivers and their potential and actual caregivers on community-based care. Refer back to the definitions at the end of the last chapter for ease of interpretation. The overlay of the life course perspective reminds us that these characteristics and relationships may differ by age and should be considered within the context of history—specifically, the year 2000, the study year. The discussion that follows highlights specific differences between the study groups using this perspective.

Life Stage and Societal Structures

One aspect of the life course perspective is the awareness that the timing of a transition (in this case, difficulty performing everyday activities without assistance) during a person's life span can have important consequences for its outcomes (George, 2002). While functional limitation is typically seen as a product of the aging process, many chronic conditions, acute diseases, and injuries result in functional limitations at midlife. Indeed, the majority of persons with disabilities are younger than 65 (Freedman, Martin, & Shoeni, 2002). In 1999 the 10 leading causes of disability among adults aged 18–64 were arthritis/rheumatism, back or spine problems, heart trouble/hardening of the arteries, lung or respiratory problems, deafness or a hearing problems, limb/extremity stiffness, mental or emotional problems, diabetes, blindness or vision problems, and stroke (Centers for

Disease Control and Prevention [CDC], 2001). Seven of the top 10 causes of disability in the United States in 2001 were the same for 21–64-year-olds and those older than 65 (Freedman et al., 2002). In 2000 approximately 20% of those aged 55–64 had activity limitations that were caused by chronic conditions (Pastor et al., 2002). This percentage rose to 26% among 65–74-year-olds and 45% among those 75 and older (Pastor et al.). The median age of detectable chronic disability is estimated to be 55 (Bruce & Fries, 2003). Clearly, functional limitation prior to retirement is a reality for many Americans.

Late middle age is a particularly vulnerable time for individuals needing help with ADLs or IADLs. This is true for three main reasons: members of the potential support group available to those in late middle age have many competing demands for their time; access to appropriate health insurance is often limited; and the safety net of federal and state services designed to provide nutrition and transportation to those in need is age-based, making most late-middle-aged people ineligible. Each of these reasons is examined in further detail next.

First, just as late-middle-aged adults with functional limitations at the time of the study were in a different stage of life compared with their older counterparts, so too were members of their social networks. While persons of late middle age were more likely to have a spouse present than older persons (U.S. Census Bureau, Public Information Office, 2001), that spouse was likely working-aged and participating in the labor force. Additionally, although middle-aged adults were more likely than older persons to have living parents, these parents may have been functionally limited themselves and unable to assist in the care of an adult child. Furthermore, children of those in late middle age were likely to be in a busy life stage themselves, limiting their ability to help functionally limited parents. If these children had actually reached adulthood, they may have been pursuing educational degrees, developing careers, forming families, and/or moving farther from loved ones.

In contrast, at the time of this study the spouses of older persons were likely to be retired and have more free time. While parental help was unavailable, older persons relied on adult children for assistance (Stone, Cafferata, & Sangl, 1987). These children were likely to be older than the children of persons in late middle age, and thus farther along in their career and family paths, potentially allowing them more flexibility with their schedules in order to assist ailing parents. A recent study of the "sandwich generation" in Canada (individuals aged 45–64 who have children under 25 living at home and who are also caring for their aging parents) found that 15% of these caregivers to aging parents reduced work hours, 20% changed work schedules, and 10% incurred a loss of income (Williams, 2004). These may not be viable options for the adult children of those in late middle age still early in their career and family formation.

Even when family support is available to those in late middle age, it may not be utilized. Indeed, compared with those 65 and older, individuals aged 50–64 have been shown to perceive less family support and greater family conflict (Turner, 1996). Literature focusing on the use of personal assistants for the severely physically disabled (i.e., individuals hired and trained directly by the care recipient to help with the personal care tasks usually performed by family members) suggests that many individuals, particularly younger adults, prefer not to rely on the assistance of family and friends (Allen & Ciambrone, 2003). Through the use of personal assistant services, loss of autonomy and burdening family members with caregiving tasks are simultaneously avoided.

Second, while informal help may be less accessible or desirable to those in late middle age, federal health care policy has virtually ignored the needs of this group. Access to appropriate health care is critical on many levels. Three include (a) primary prevention to maintain overall health, (b) accessibility to treatment for acute episodes in order to protect against negative chronic outcomes, and (c) assistance with maintenance of chronic conditions to prevent further decline or secondary conditions. But while health insurance is key to both health maintenance and rehabilitation, individuals in late middle age are at high risk for lacking any type of insurance (Pol et al., 2000). Medicare, which covers the cost of certain home health services and durable medical equipment, begins at age 65. Part A coverage is available to some who are disabled prior to the age of 65, although many in need do not pass strict eligibility criteria. In order to receive Medicare benefits prior to age 65, an individual must be eligible to receive and have received social security disability benefits for 24 months. This requires that she or he has worked at least 20 of the last 40 quarters, and is now judged to be so limited that she or he cannot work for at least the next year (Centers for Medicare and Medicaid Services [CMS], n.d.; Moon, 1996). Medicaid is only available to individuals in late middle age who meet both strict financial and disability criteria, and benefits vary considerably by state (Iezonni, 2003).

Given that most middle-aged adults, even those with functional limitations, do not meet both financial and disability criteria, private health insurance is the dominant source of insurance for this group. Private insurance covers little in terms of chronic care needs and is often dependent upon one's (or one's spouse's) continued presence in the workforce. Not surprisingly, working-aged adults with functional limitations are less likely than those without to have any form of private health insurance (LaPlante, 1993; McCarty & Levine, 1999).

Finally, federal and state aging services that provide nutrition and transportation have helped to alleviate some of the need of frail elders, but have done little for middle-aged adults (Administration on Aging [AoA], n.d.; Allen & Mor, 1997). Programs such as Meals on Wheels and RIDE serve thousands yearly, but because they are organized by Area Agencies on Aging rather than disability-based groups, eligibility criteria include an age cutoff of 60 (AoA, 2004). Ultimately, therefore, individuals in late middle age without informal help or adequate health insurance must go without help or rely upon their own financial resources to purchase it. Here again, they may be at a distinct disadvantage compared with the older population. Many who have yet to see their full earnings potential may be forced to leave the labor force, perhaps greatly reducing any pension that they would have been eligible for had they worked to normal retirement age (Freedman et al., 2002). They may still be supporting dependent children, or they may have become disabled early in life and have experienced the cumulative economic disadvantage of being disabled throughout adulthood (Wang, 2005).

Cohort Differences

In addition to life stage differences, there are substantial cohort differences between individuals in late middle age and their older counterparts. This study's older old group (previously defined as 75 and older) entered old age at a unique point in American history. They benefited from medical and public health advances that increased their life spans and reduced their years of morbidity (National Institute on Aging [NIA], 1999). As a group, they were better-off financially than those who came before. At the time, the poverty rate of 9.7% in 1999 for people 65 and older was the lowest for this group ever measured by the U.S. Census Bureau's Public Information Office (2001). On average, they had three children who survived past the age of 40 (Glasgow, 2000) and had high rates of marriage and low rates of divorce. They benefited from generous social security pensions and near-universal access to Medicare. These benefits helped to change retirement ages. While in the 1940s half of all men over age 64 worked, by 1997 only 16% of such men worked (Levy, 1998).

A desire for independent living increased in this generation as well, perhaps due to greater financial autonomy or changes in values (Crimmins & Ingegneri, 1990; Kramarow, 1995; Macunovich, Easterlin, Schaeffer, & Crimmons, 1995; Ruggles, 1995). However, even with this desire for independence, a clear pattern of intergenerational exchange in time of need has been evident (Silverstein, 1995). The current older old group members have been able to help their adult children in times of financial and housing needs (Hogan, Eggebeen, & Clogg, 1993; Speare & Avery, 1993). In return, their children have provided them with assistance when they become frail (Stone et al., 1987). In short, they have benefited from the demographic and economic transformations of modernity, but did not participate in the family revolutions that followed (Goldscheider, 1990).

The experiences of individuals in late middle age in 2000 have and will continue to differ from those of older persons. They were at the forefront of the "family revolutions," experiencing later childbearing and reduced overall fertility. They experienced greater divorce and childlessness than their older counterparts (Goldscheider, 1990; Kreider & Simmons, 2003). They were more racially and ethnically diverse than previous generations (Hobbs & Stoops, 2002). Their households, and especially those of their adult children, relied more heavily upon the earnings of two individuals, as real wages have declined over the past 30 years (Harrison & Bluestone, 1998; Levy, 1998). Importantly, the children of this cohort, particularly those born since 1966, are aging during a time of great economic uncertainty, straining their ability to secure even their own futures (Karner, 2001). It is unclear how this will affect their ability to assist functionally dependent parents in their time of need (Karner). At the same time, adults in late middle age are entering the years immediately preceding retirement amidst an endangered Medicare system, risking financial failure in the absence of sweeping reform. They are forced more than the current older generation to consider how they will support themselves for potentially 20 or more years past the traditional retirement age of 65.

Who Provides Care

Now that differences between the characteristics of the late-middle-aged adults and their older counterparts, their potential helpers, and their access to federal safety nets have been highlighted, we next turn to what we currently know about community-based care. This information is predominantly based on the study of older persons. An extensive body of research affirms that families provide the bulk of care to frail elders (e.g., Jette et al., 1992; Kemper, 1988; Stone et al., 1987, Wolff & Kasper, 2006). Spouses, if available, are the most likely to provide care, followed by adult daughters (Messeri, Silverstein, & Litwak, 1993; Wolff & Kasper). Other kin (e.g., adult siblings) and nonkin provide much less hands-on assistance to individuals with functional limitations. When formal (i.e., paid) assistance is used by elders, it acts mainly as a supplement to existing informal care, rather than as a substitution for it (Penning, 2002; Tennstedt, Harrow, & Crawford, 1996). These findings support Litwak's task-specificity model of care (Litwak, 1985).

Gender Differences

Though women are entering the workforce at increasingly steady rates, and dual-earner families are common, women are still considered the primary caregivers to family members in need (Collins, Schoen, & Joseph, 1999). Men do assume the role of caregiver, but they do so less frequently than women. Sons, for instance, are more likely to provide care to elderly parents when there are no daughters available. Men also provide fewer hours of care overall, and less intense care than women (Horowitz, 1985; Neal, Ingersoll-Dayton, & Starrels, 1997; Stoller, 1990). Male caregivers are more likely to provide assistance with less personal IADL tasks than with ADLs (Stoller). Compared with men, women are less likely to name their spouse as their primary caregiver and more likely to rely on others to supplement their husband's help (Allen, Goldscheider, & Ciambrone, 1999; Allen, 1994).

Cultural Differences

Cultural differences, specifically racial and ethnic differences, in social networks have been widely documented—but due to limitations in sample sizes and analytic methodology, they have not always shown consistent results. Despite the notion that Blacks in particular benefit from a wider social network by incorporating fictive kin (i.e., individuals not related by blood or marriage but still considered family; Cantor, Brennan, & Sainz, 1994; Stewart, 2007), Black and Hispanic social networks tend to be smaller than those of Whites (Ajrouch et al., 2001; Roschelle, 1997). Strength of ties between family members also differ. While Whites showed the strongest bonds between parent and child, a study of individuals 85 and older found that Blacks placed greater emphasis on the bonds between siblings than did Whites (Johnson, 2000).

These differences are reflected in the caregiving literature that shows differences in the type, structure, and amount of care across race and ethnicity (e.g., Dilworth-Anderson, Williams, & Gibson, 2002; Stommel, Given, & Given, 1998; Wallace, Levy-Storms, Kington, & Andersen, 1998). For instance, Whites are more likely than Blacks to receive all of their care from a sole individual, rather than share caregiving tasks across two or more people (Stommel et al., 1998). But, while Blacks may have greater numbers of caregivers overall, they are more likely than Whites to receive no care at all and inadequate amounts of care when care is provided (Lima & Allen, 2001). Alternatively, Hispanics are as likely as Whites to have a caregiver, but more likely to receive inadequate care when care is provided (Lima & Allen).

Risks and Consequences of Inadequate Care

As DeJong and Brannont (1998) pointed out, studies of personal care that include nonelderly persons are generally based on the need for, rather than the utilization of, such care. Results point to differences in levels of unmet need that may be attributable to the life stage and cohort differences between late-middle-aged and elderly adults described earlier (Allen & Mor, 1997; LaPlante et al., 2004; Lima & Allen, 2001). Allen and Mor found that increased levels of unmet need for IADLs and transportation help for respondents less than 65 compared with 65 and older were explained by financial problems among the younger group.

This finding was further supported by Allen and Mor (1997), who compared differences in the levels of unmet need for assistance with transportation and nutrition services between the working-aged and elderly adults to levels of support services used. They found that the lower level of unmet need among elderly persons compared with working-aged adults was almost perfectly complimented by an increased level of use of state-supported transportation and nutrition services. What little is known about the care networks of working-aged individuals is that they rely less upon formal services than their elderly counterparts (LaPlante, Harrington, & Kang, 2002).

In addition, racial/ethnic minority status and divorce are both positively associated with unmet need for care, as is a lack of Medicare and/or Medicaid coverage (Lima & Allen, 2001). Those who perceive their support network to be less resilient to their needs, and those who have fewer children living nearby are also at greater risk of unmet need for care (Mor, Allen, Siegel, & Houts, 1992).

Both regional and national studies of adults with disabling conditions have found that fully one-third to one-half of people experience one or more adverse consequences associated with inadequate care in a month's time that have implications for health status and service utilization. Adverse consequences include falls, burns, going hungry, inability to follow special diets, weight loss, dehydration, wetting or soiling self, missing physician appointments, and depression (Allen & Mor, 1997; Desai, Lentzner, & Weeks, 2001; Komisar, Feder, & Kasper, 2005; LaPlante et al., 2004). Inadequate care is also associated with hospitalization and emergency room use (Long, King, & Couglin, 2005–2006; Sands et al., 2006).

There is evidence suggesting that public policies can reduce unmet need in populations with long-term care needs. A survey of dual enrollees in Medicare and Medicaid in six states revealed high levels of unmet need overall (58% of respondents with long-term care needs). However, lower levels of unmet need for ADL assistance were observed in states in which a higher proportion of people received paid care (Komisar et al., 2005).

State and federally funded services can clearly help those who have access to them.

Summary

As we have previously mentioned, most of what the research community knows about the care networks of individuals with limitations in function comes from research on the elderly population. The aforementioned descriptions demonstrate, however, that the life courses of those in late middle age and their older counterparts at the beginning of the 21st century were quite distinct. Researchers cannot assume that the care networks of these groups function similarly.

Within the life course perspective, requiring help in midlife versus late life involves an entirely different set of circumstances. One basic premise of this study is that there are life stage differences, not only between the young and older respondents with ADL and/or IADL difficulties, but also between the members of the respondents' support networks that limit the number of hours of care received by individuals in late middle age with functional limitations compared with those who are young old or older old. In the analyses to follow, life stage differences were quantified primarily by examining differences in the characteristics of members of the respondents' social support groups and more narrowly defined care networks. For example, considering Litwak's proximity dimension, we expected to find that the spouses of those in late middle age compared with those of their older counterparts were more likely to be working outside of the home and have competing care responsibilities for parents and/or dependent children. These characteristics would make them less available to provide large amounts of care compared with their older counterparts. Potential child caregivers for late-middle-aged adults, likewise, were likely to be younger, have younger children of their own to care for, and be in a less secure financial state (as measured in part by home ownership and hours of work) than the child caregivers of older old adults. Speaking not only to Litwak's proximity dimension but also to the level of commitment dimension, younger adults may feel less of a commitment to help their functionally limited parent given their own needs to raise young children and foster their careers. Functionally limited adults, likewise, may differ on the social role dimension depending on their age, such that those in late middle age may be less inclined to ask their children for help because it is not part of the normal aging process. Older persons may view this help as a typical role reversal between parent and child that comes with aging. Where they once cared for their children, now their children are caring for them. We expected that these potential life stage differences would contribute to differences both in the likelihood of the receipt of any care and in hours of care that were received.

Cohort differences also existed between the age groups in this study. The young were more likely to be of minority status, have reduced overall fertility, and be divorced compared with their older counterparts (Downs, 2003; Hobbs & Stoops, 2002). All of these factors associated with individuals in late middle age are also associated with higher rates of disability and/or reduced availability of care (Freedman et al., 2002; Lima & Allen, 2001); this is suggestive that the young would be in greater peril than the older old group in terms of receipt of care. Therefore, we controlled for cohort characteristics in all multivariate analyses.

HYPOTHESES

Thus, based on demonstrated differences in the life course of the three age groups under study, we expected to find that the community-based care experiences of individuals in late middle age and perhaps those who were young old with functional limitations would differ greatly from their older old counterparts. First, we hypothesized that individuals in late middle age with functional limitations would be less likely to receive any help with their limitations compared with their older counterparts. Among those who did receive at least a minimum of help, we expected to find that the composition of the care networks would differ across age groups. We hypothesized that the care networks of individuals in late middle age would be more likely to include spouses and nonkin than their older counterparts, but less likely to include children and paid help. Perhaps more important than the composition of the care networks, however, we expected that individuals in late middle age would receive fewer hours of care, not only from their primary caregivers, but also from their entire care networks compared with their older counterparts.

We also tested for the possibility that certain characteristics operated differently by age. For example, given that divorce rates have now been high for many years, it was possible that the negative consequences of divorce on family support had lessened such that being divorced did not reduce the availability or amount of care for younger cohorts as much as it did for older cohorts. It was also possible that individuals in late middle age incorporated the use of formal services into their care networks differently from older age groups. Though older age groups used formal services as a supplement to informal care by family members, perhaps individuals in late middle age who had access to formal services used them as a substitute for some hours of care from their informal members. These and other possibilities were examined throughout the analyses.

Chapter 3

Data and Methods

Data Source

The primary data set for this study was the Health and Retirement Study (HRS), which is sponsored by the National Institute on Aging (grant number NIA U01AG009740) and is conducted by the University of Michigan. The study began in 1992 with a national sample of adults in the contiguous United States born between 1931 and 1941, representative of those aged 51–61 living in the community. Respondents have been followed every 2 years. Parallel to this, its sister study, the Assets and Health Dynamics of the Oldest Old (AHEAD), began in 1993 and included a representative sample of community-dwelling individuals aged 70 and older (born in or before 1923). Again, respondents were followed every 2 years. In 1998 the two studies joined while at the same time adding two new age cohorts to the study in order to make the HRS henceforth representative of the population aged 50 and older. These additions included the younger War Babies, born between 1942 and 1947, and the filler group between the original HRS and AHEAD cohorts, the Children of the Depression Era (CODA), born between 1924 and 1930. The survey continues to be fielded every 2 years and remains representative of the population aged 50 and older, being weighted based on the survey year's Current Population Survey. Due to data availability specific to the research topic, we used the 2000 wave for our study.

We also made use of version D of RAND's longitudinal file, an independent data file consisting of the first five waves of data and providing numerous summary variables created by RAND and derived from the original data files.

HRS Response Rates

Initial response rates for the four sample cohorts (HRS, AHEAD, War Babies, and CODA) differed due to differences in their recruitment methods. The initial HRS cohort had an initial response rate of 81.7% in 1992, AHEAD had an initial rate of 80.4% in 1993, CODA had a rate of 72.4% in 1998, and War Babies had a rate of 70.1% in 1998. Nevertheless, for respondents who were successfully interviewed in the first wave of a study cohort, there was a high level of reinterview, with each cohort having a reinterview rate of over 91% for each successive wave. Therefore, overall attrition was low. Comprehensive information regarding sample design and response rates can be found at the HRS Web site (http://hrsonline.isr.umich.edu/intro/sho_uinfo.php?hfyle=sample&xtyp=2). Appropriate weights and statistical techniques were used throughout to make the overall sample representative of the population aged 50 and older for any particular survey year.

Advantages of the HRS

The HRS was ideal for a study of this kind. First, the consolidation in 1998 of the original HRS and AHEAD cohorts, as well as the addition of the filler cohorts, made it possible to compare our age groups of interest. Second, because a major focus of the HRS is to examine intergenerational exchanges of time and money, it has extensive information on vertical family members. This data set, like no others, allows the researcher to examine not only the actual network characteristics of individuals who receive care but also the characteristics of their set of potential helpers, the social network. There is extensive information on the existence and availability of children and parents, as well as the competing demands that these individuals may face when deciding whether or not, and how much, they can help a relative in need.

Unlike other surveys designed to study topics relating to community-based care, it also has extensive spousal information. In fact, we had as much information on the health and sociodemographic characteristics of the spouse, a potential helper, as we did on the person with functional limitations because within married households both individuals were asked to complete the survey.

Limitations of the HRS

While the HRS is the premier data source for a study of this kind, there were a number of limitations surrounding its use. First, although it would have been ideal to begin a cohort study by comparing 51–61-year-old adults in 1992 to their 2002 counterparts, the 1992 survey did not ask about the care networks of individuals who might need assistance with ADLs or IADLs. Therefore, the HRS was unable at the time of these analyses to support formal analyses to examine differences in hours of care that may have resulted from true cohort differences.

Second, at the time of this study, the HRS lacked a direct measure of unmet need. This omission was problematic for this study for two reasons. First, without it we assumed that respondents with the same level of casemix who had fewer hours of care than their counterparts had unmet need. We based this assumption on the work of LaPlante et al. (2004), who investigated the association between unmet need and reported hours of help received in the 1994–1995 National Health Interview Survey's Disability Supplement (NHIS-D), controlling for level of need, living arrangements, and other factors that might be expected to differ between persons with met and unmet need. They found that respondents with unmet need in two or more ADLs had a shortfall of 16.6 hours of help per week compared with respondents whose needs were met (LaPlante et al.).

A second issue regarding the absence of a measure of unmet need was that there was a substantial proportion of people who reported difficulty in performing at least one ADL and/or IADL but had no help, suggesting that they may have had unmet need. However, estimates from the 1994–1995 Disability Supplement to the National Health Interview Survey, which included comprehensive measures of unmet need and its consequences, indicated that only a small minority of people who had difficulty performing daily living activities but did not receive help reported needing it. Among 1934 noninstitutionalized adults aged 50 and over in the NHIS-D who reported difficulty with at least one ADL or IADL but received no help, only 11.4% (220) stated that they needed help, that is, that they had unmet need (unpublished estimates). Clearly, while these respondents were experiencing difficulty performing daily living activities, they were still able to do so independently. Previous work by Lima and Allen (2001) found that such respondents were less severely impaired than those who had no help and said they needed it, and the latter respondents, in turn, were less severely impaired than respondents who received help but reported it was not enough. Thus, the absence of a measure of unmet need from this data set was a shortcoming but not a major concern in this regard.

Third, at the time of this study, the HRS inquired about neither the onset of the functional limitation nor when the respondent began receiving help. It would have been useful to know if the respondent had been receiving help for months or for years, as the care network may have evolved over time. However, we were able to examine the number of years since diagnosis of individuals' primary disabling condition for the approximately one-half of the sample who had been enrolled as part of the original HRS cohort. Results indicated surprisingly similar lengths of time for all age groups, that is, 13 years for the youngest (50–64) and oldest (75 and older) age groups, and 14 years for the intermediate (65–74) group. Also, in our full analytic sample, roughly similar and relatively small (i.e., <10%) proportions of respondents across age groups reported diagnosis of eight of the most common chronic conditions (psychological problems, arthritis, high blood pressure, cancer, diabetes, lung disease, heart problems, and stroke) within the past 2 years. Thus, it did not appear that length of disability varied widely by age, and that the majority of sample members in all age groups had lived with their conditions for a substantial period of time. This may be due to the fact that we selected only those respondents who had become functionally impaired by their condition, which generally occurs over time as a disease progresses.

Study Sample

In 1998 the HRS and AHEAD combined, marking the first survey round that allowed for comparisons between the young and old.

Due to data limitations in the measurement of hours of care in 1998, we used the 2000 survey. A total of 18,149 individuals representative of the civilian noninstitutionalized U.S. population aged 50 and older participated in the HRS in 2000. Of this number, 4,000 people (22% of the total sample) reported having difficulty performing at least one ADL or IADL. This subgroup constituted the analytic sample for examining the receipt of care. Of the 4,000, 2,259 received assistance with at least one ADL or IADL in the month prior to the survey. This subgroup constituted the analytic sample for examining the composition of the care networks and the hours of care received.

MEASURES

The variables of interest can be grouped into the following categories: dependent variables, sociodemographic characteristics of the respondent, respondent casemix, characteristics of the respondent's social network, characteristics of the caregiving network, and characteristics of the two most prevalent primary caregivers—spouses and children. Summary table 3.1 is provided. We used many of the independent variables listed to describe the social networks and narrower support networks of the respondents, but we did not use them in subsequent analyses to model hours of care.

Dependent Variables

There were three sets of dependent variables: whether or not any help was received, the composition of the care network, and hours of care in the last month. Respondents were asked a series of questions regarding ADLs and IADLs. If the respondent stated having difficulty in at least one ADL or IADL, the respondent was further asked if she or he received assistance from anyone with that particular activity. The relationship of

TABLE 3.1. Variables, descriptions, and operationalizations.

Type	Variable(s)	Description	Operationalization
Dependent Variables	Receipt of care	Whether or not the respondent reported receiving care from one or more persons in the month prior to the survey	1 = Yes 0 = No
	Composition of care	Based on number of caregivers, gender, and relationship of caregivers to respondent	Number of adult children providing care—continuous Presence of Spouse (1/0) Nonrelative (1/0) Formal Care (1/0) Secondary help (1/0)
	Hours of care in last month	Respondents who stated that they received help from 1 or more people in the last month with ADLs or IADLs were asked how many days in the last month each caregiver assisted him/her. They were then asked how many hours per day, on the days they were helped, did that caregiver help. For this measure, hours are summed across all caregivers.	Hours in past month were truncated at 720 (i.e., 24 hours per day, everyday) and then logged Separate measures for total care, and care provided by primary caregiver

(*continued on next page*)

TABLE 3.1. *(continued)*

Type	Variable(s)	Description	Operationalization
Independent Variables			
Sociodemographic Characteristics of the Survey Respondent	Gender		1 = Male 0 = Female
	Age	The classification of age groups in this study emphasizes potential differences across life stage and cohort.	1 = 50–64 2 = 65–74 3 = 75+
	Marital status	Current marital status	1 = Married/partnered 2 = Divorced/separated 3 = Widowed 4 = Never married
	Race/ethnicity	A race/ethnicity variable is possible due to the oversampling of Blacks and Hispanics in this dataset. Other race/ethnicities are too infrequent to further categorize.	1 = non-Hispanic White 2 = non-Hispanic Black 3 = Hispanic 4 = Other
	Education	The low prevalence of any education beyond high school among the oldest age group precludes a more detailed variable form.	1 = Less than high school 2 = High school diploma 3 = More than high school
	Insurance	Insurance status at time of interview; inclusion in more than one category is possible	Medicare (1/0) Medicaid (1, 0) Private (1, 0) Uninsured (1, 0)

	Income	Total household income includes respondent and spouse earnings, household capital, respondent and spouse pensions, respondent and spouse social security disability income (SSDI) or supplemental security income (SSI), respondent and spouse income from social security retirement, respondent and spouse income from unemployment or worker's compensation, respondent and spouse income from other government transfers, and all other reported household income.	Quintiles based on general population aged 50+
	Work status	An indicator of whether or not the respondent is currently working for pay	1 = Yes 0 = No
	Living arrangement	An indicator of whether or not the respondent lives alone or with others	1 = Lives alone 0 = Lives with others
Respondent Case Mix	Functional Impairment	Separate counts of the number of ADLs and IADLs with which a respondent reports difficulty. ADLs include bathing, walking, eating, toileting,	Continuous variables ADL: Range 0–6 IADL: Range 0–5

(*continued on next page*)

TABLE 3.1. *(continued)*

Type	Variable(s)	Description	Operationalization
		getting into and out of bed, and dressing and are derived from the Activities of Daily Living Scale (Katz & Akpom, 1976). IADLs include managing money, preparing meals, getting groceries, using the telephone, and taking medications and are based on the Instrumental Activities of Daily Living Scale (Lawton, 1971).	
	Overall health	Self-reported health status scored on a continuum based on work by Diehr and colleagues (2002, 1995) who found that scoring the responses as 96, 93, 75, 45, and 19 yields the estimated percent probability that a person will be healthy 2 years in the future.	Continuous measure Excellent = 96 Very good = 93 Good = 75 Fair = 45 Poor = 19
	Cognitive impairment	Based on following reasons for proxy respondent: (b) may have some cognitive limitations but could probably do the interview; (c) has cognitive limitations that prevent him/her from being interviewed; and (d) this is a cognitive interview; that is, respondent started to do an interview but received a low TICS score in section C.	1 = Cognitive impairment 0 = None

Wheelchair use	Respondents were asked whether or not they used any assistive devices to help them walk across a room or get out of bed. Wheelchairs were one of the options.	1 = Used wheelchair 0 = Did not
Fatigue	An indicator of whether or not the respondent considered him/herself to be extremely fatigued or exhausted in the 2 weeks prior to the survey	1 = Yes 0 = No
BMI	Body mass index was recoded to indicate whether a person was underweight (BMI ≤ 18.5), normal/Obese (18.5 < BMI < 40), or morbidly obese (BMI ≥ 40)	1 = Underweight 2 = Normal/obese 3 = Morbidly obese
Nights in hospital	An indicator of the number of nights a respondent spent in the hospital between surveys, or in the 2 years prior to the survey if this was the respondent's first survey	Count
Bed days	An indicator of the number of days spent in bed over the past month	Count
Medical conditions	An indicator of the number of medical conditions the respondent reported of the following: arthritis, lung disease, heart problems, high blood pressure,	Count

(*continued on next page*)

TABLE 3.1. *(continued)*

Type	Variable(s)	Description	Operationalization
		stroke, cancer, psychological disorder, and diabetes	
	Psychological disorder	Presence of this particular medical condition	1 = Yes 0 = No
Characteristics of the Respondent's Social Network	Adult daughters	Number/presence of daughters aged 18 and older	Count and dichotomous measure of presence of any 1 = Yes 0 = No
	Adult sons	Number/presence of sons aged 18 and older	Same as above
	Living brothers	Number/presence of living brothers	Same as above
	Living sisters	Number/presence of living sisters	Same as above
	Living parents	Number/presence of living parents/-in-laws	Same as above
	Anyone in network	An indicator of whether or not the respondent had at least one of the following individuals in his network: other household member or nonresident children, siblings, and/or parents	1 = Yes 0 = No
Characteristics of the Respondent's Care Network	Size of Informal network	Number of family and nonrelatives who assisted the respondent with ADLs and/or IADLs in the past month	Count
	Formal care	Presence of at least one formal caregiver in network	1 = Yes 0 = No

	Overall structure of care network	Combination of caregiver types	1 = Spouse only 2 = Informal only (may include spouse) 3 = Formal only 4 = Both informal and informal
	Relation to the respondent	Relation of the primary caregiver to the respondent	1 = Spouse 2 = Child 3 = Other relative 4 = Nonrelative 5 = Formal
Characteristics of Spouse Primary Caregiver	Work status	Current work status	Two measures 1 = Currently working for pay 0 = Not working
		Hours measured per week	1 = Working less than 20 hours 2 = Working between 20 and 39 hours 3 = Working 40 hours 4 = Working more than 40 hours 5 = Not working
	Functional status	Number of ADL difficulties and number of IADL difficulties	Counts
	Receipt of care	Indicator of whether or not the spouse caregiver is also receiving help with his or her own ADL/IADL limitations	1 = Yes 0 = No
	Gender		1 = Female 0 = Male

(continued on next page)

TABLE 3.1. *(continued)*

Type	Variable(s)	Description	Operationalization
	Other caregiving responsibilities	Indicator of whether or not the spouse caregiver is also providing care to children under 18 years old or to ailing parents	1 = Yes 0 = No
Characteristics of Child Primary Caregivers	Gender		1 = Male 0 = Female
	Work status	Current work status	1 = >30 hours per week 2 = <30 hours per week 3 = Does not work 4 = Missing
	Home ownership		1 = Yes 0 = No
	Has children		1 = Yes 0 = No
	Currently married		1 = Yes 0 = No
	Living arrangement	The proximity of the child caregiver to the respondent	1 = Lives with the respondent 2 = Lives within 10 miles of respondent 3 = Lives farther than 10 miles from respondent
	Age		Continuous measure

the caregiver to the respondent was assessed so that the first set of dependent variables (whether or not any help is received) distinguishes between informal and formal help.

The second set of dependent variables examined the composition of the care network. Age differences were examined for the number of children in the care network, as well as the presence of a spouse, nonrelative, formal care, or any secondary help.

Respondents who stated that they received help from one or more people in the last month with ADLs or IADLs were asked how many days in that month each caregiver assisted him or her and how many hours per day. The third set of dependent variables examined total hours of care in the past month and hours from the primary caregiver only. Subanalyses were conducted on hours provided by spousal primary caregivers and child primary caregivers.

Though the use of time diaries is considered a better method of measuring time spent in particular activities than survey recall methods, time diaries are often cumbersome, time-consuming, and generally impractical for many studies (van den Berg & Spauwen, 2006). The HRS, like other major surveys involving informal caregiving, such as the National Long Term Care Survey and the National Longitudinal Study of Aging, made use of the recall method as previously described. Though this method may suffer somewhat from recall bias and overestimation (van den Berg & Spauwen), LaPlante et al. (2004) supplied face validity to the measure by documenting a relationship between unmet need for care and shortfall of hours of care received among individuals who report two or more ADL limitations. No studies have been conducted to determine whether recall bias in the report of caregiving hours differs by age.

The total number of hours was the sum of hours across all caregivers. In order to deal with outliers on the high end, we truncated responses that were the equivalent of more than 24 hours per day of care for 30 days to 24 hours per day.[1] This occurred when, for example, an individual reported receiving around-the-clock care from two or more individuals. The variable was further transformed into natural log hours since the distribution of hours was heavily skewed, and it is common within the literature to use the natural logarithm of hours of care (e.g., Katz, Kabeto, & Langa, 2000; LaPlante et al., 2002) in order to conduct ordinary least squares analysis. Similar measures of hours of care by the primary caregiver, the spouse primary caregiver and the child primary caregiver were also used.

Six percent of caregivers were missing a measure of hours of care. This was possible in two ways: when the respondent did not provide the number of days per month that the caregiver helped out, or alternatively, when the respondent did not provide the number of hours per day. Though this occurred in only 6% of caregivers, it represented 8% of respondents for whom at least one of their caregivers was missing information. Because hours for every caregiver in an individual's network was critical in order to measure total hours of care, we imputed the missing values rather than be forced to eliminate these individuals from the analyses altogether and lose valuable information. We employed multiple hot-deck imputation, a single imputation technique, whereby the missing and nonmissing values for the variable of interest are stratified by one or more characteristics and missing values are replaced by random draws taken from the nonmissing values within a particular stratum (Kalton & Kasprzyk, 1986). We stratified by age group and relationship of the caregiver to the respondent. Though multiple imputation techniques are generally considered preferable to single imputation techniques because they allow for uncertainty and adjust the standard errors accordingly (Rubin, 1996; for an exception, see Paul, Mason,

McCaffrey, & Fox, 2003), at the time of the analyses the multiple imputation procedure in Stata, the statistical software package used for this study, did not support the use of survey procedures, which were needed due to the complex survey design.

Once imputation was complete, we assigned primary caregiver status to the person who provided the most hours of care in the month prior to the survey. When a tie occurred among two or more caregivers within the same network (this occurred in approximately 5% of cases), the following rules were employed:

1. If the respondent named one of the people in the tie as the main helper with ADL tasks, then that person was designated the primary caregiver; else
2. if the respondent named one of the people in the tie as the main helper with IADL tasks, then that person was designated the primary caregiver; else
3. if the respondent named one of the people in the tie as the main helper with managing money, then that person was designated the primary caregiver.
4. If none of the above conditions were met, then the primary caregiver was arbitrarily assigned. This occurred in less than 1% of 2,259 care networks.

Sociodemographic Characteristics of the Respondent

The primary characteristic of importance in this category was age. In studies of care utilization or need, researchers rarely consider the life course and cohort consequences of age. Age is either treated as a continuous measure or grouped into large categories, usually 18–64 and 65 and older (e.g., Agree & Freedman, 2003; LaPlante et al., 2004; Lima & Allen, 2001; Allen & Mor, 1997). In this study, age was divided into three groups: late middle age (50–64), the young old (65–74), and the older old (75 and older). The youngest group consisted of members younger than the traditional retirement age who were more likely than older groups to have dependent children, and for the most part they did not qualify for the aging services mentioned previously. The next group, the young old, were past the traditional retirement age, more likely than the oldest group to have a living spouse, and if they had children, these children were likely to be mid-career with dependent children of their own. Finally, members of the oldest group were the least likely to have a living spouse, but the most likely to have adult children in the position to assist them.

There were a number of characteristics that differed by age that were also associated with the receipt of care. They were gender, marital status, race/ethnicity, education, insurance, and income. We describe the reasons for considering each next.

While women have larger care networks, they receive less help from their spouses than do men (Allen, 1994; Katz et al., 2000). They are equally likely as men to receive some care, but more likely than men to receive inadequate care when care is provided (Lima & Allen, 2001). In addition, because of gender differences in longevity, women comprise a greater portion of the older old group than other age groups.

Those who are divorced or who have never been married are less likely to receive care compared with either the widowed or currently married (Lima & Allen, 2001; Pezzin & Schone, 1999). Furthermore, the divorced are more likely than other groups to receive inadequate care when care is provided (Lima & Allen). In this study, we divided marital status into four groups: married/partnered, divorced/separated, widowed, and never married. Preliminary comparisons indicated that there were no significant differences in care receipt between married and partnered couples, and so we did not distinguish between them, but rather refer to them as "married" throughout the remainder of the analyses. We also did not distinguish same-sex couples, as there were only a handful in our sample, nor did we deliberately exclude them. If they referred to themselves as married or partnered, they were grouped as such.

We previously described cultural differences in social networks and the receipt of care. Because our focus was on life course differences in care and because the percentage of racial and ethnic minorities differs greatly by age group (Hobbs & Stoops, 2002), race/ethnicity was controlled for with four categories: non-Hispanic White, non-Hispanic Black, Hispanic, and Other.

One study that included adults 18 and older showed no association between educational attainment and care received (e.g., see Lima & Allen, 2001). Another examining the elder population only found that lower levels of education were significantly related to unmet need of care (Desai et al., 2001). Therefore, it was important to consider it here, particularly given age differences in education levels. We divided education into three categories: less than high school, high school, and more than high school.

At least in studies using data collected prior to changes in the Balanced Budget Acts of 1997 and 1999 that significantly reduced home care covered by Medicare, the receipt of public health insurance (either Medicare or Medicaid) significantly reduced one's risk of going without care when care was needed (Lima & Allen, 2001; Wallace et al., 1998). This study controlled primarily for Medicaid because the receipt of Medicare is tied closely to age. However, Medicare is examined descriptively in chapter 4.

Finally, income level was controlled. Approximately 20% of home care to older persons is paid for out-of-pocket, and another 42% by Medicare (Congressional Budget Office, 2004).

Out-of-pocket expenses may be even higher for individuals in late middle age who are not universally covered by Medicare. LaPlante et al. (2002) found that higher levels of income were associated with receiving paid care. RAND has developed summary measures of income from the HRS. This study employed a five-category measure of total income, which included respondent and spouse earnings, household capital, respondent and spouse pensions, respondent and spouse social security disability income (SSDI) or supplemental security income (SSI), respondent and spouse income from social security retirement, respondent and spouse income from unemployment or worker's compensation, respondent and spouse income from other government transfers, and all other reported household income. Similar to the technique used by Katz et al. (2000), total household income was used as a five-category variable that broke the total household income for the entire HRS sample (representing the general noninstitutionalized population aged 50 and older) into quintiles.

Respondent Casemix

The amount of care received is invariably at least partly related to the amount of care that is needed. While a direct measure of need was not available in this survey, there were a number of useful variables that reflected the respondents' physical level of functioning.

First, we measured functional impairment with two variables: the number of ADLs (range 0–6) and IADLs (range 0–5) the respondent reports difficulty performing. ADLs included dressing, walking across a room, bathing, getting out of bed, eating, and toileting (Katz & Akpom, 1976). IADLs included preparing meals, going grocery shopping, using the phone, managing medications, and managing money (Lawton, 1971).

We also controlled for self-reported health status and cognitive impairment. Respondents reported their general health as being excellent, very good, good, fair, or poor. Diehr et al. (1995, 2002) found that scoring these responses as 96, 93, 75, 45, and 19, respectively, and using the overall measure as a continuous variable, yields the estimated percent probability that a person will be healthy 2 years in the future. We used this continuum in our analyses.

Individuals who are cognitively impaired often require more time-consuming assistance. Indeed, caregivers of individuals with dementia provide more hours of care than do caregivers for those without dementia (Ory, Hoffman, Yee, Tennstedt, & Schulz, 1999). In addition, cognitive impairment increases dramatically with age, particularly after 65 (Lindsay & Anderson, 2004). We therefore controlled for cognitive impairment in the analyses. The specific measure used was based on a rating given by the interviewer as the reason for a proxied interview. The responses were the following: (a) no reason to think the respondent has any cognitive limitations; (b) may have some cognitive limitations but could probably do the interview; (c) has cognitive limitations that prevent him or her from being interviewed; and (d) this is a cognitive interview, that is, the respondent started to do an interview but received a low TICS score in Section C. For this study, a respondent was considered cognitively impaired if answers of (b), (c), or (d) were given.

We controlled for use of a wheelchair, whether or not the respondent was extremely fatigued or exhausted in the past 2 weeks, and whether or not the respondent was underweight (defined as having a BMI less than or equal to 18.5) or morbidly obese (defined as having a BMI greater than 40). The use of more complex assistive devices, such as wheelchairs compared with canes, is a function of disability severity

(Allen, Foster, & Berg, 2001). Extreme fatigue and whether or not the individual is underweight served as crude proxies for a measure of frailty, which in itself cannot be measured in the HRS, but which is related to a greater likelihood of concurrent medical conditions and decreased survival (Klein, Klein, Knudston, & Lee, 2005). Obesity is comorbid with disability and may be associated with reduced hours of care compared with those who are not obese (CDC, 2002; Resnik, Lapane & Allen, 2005).

We also controlled for two additional quality of life indicators: the number of nights a respondent spent in the hospital in the 2 years prior to the survey, as well as the number of times in the month prior to the interview that the respondent spent more than half of the day in bed due to a health problem.

Finally, although respondents were asked about the presence of a number of medical conditions, we only specifically controlled for the presence of psychological disorders. Most of the conditions asked about in the HRS are naturally correlated with age, but in themselves say nothing about one's functional/health status that is important to needing assistance that is not already captured in the other aforementioned variables. If a medical condition is going to lead to the need for assistance, it is going to do so through the bodily limitations it imposes. In fact, controlling for them would potentially mask, rather than identify, a possible age effect. The presence of a psychological disorder is different from other conditions, however, in that it has historically been stigmatizing to be labeled with a psychological disorder—and this stigma may affect the availability of care (Angermeyer, Beck, Dietrich, & Holzinger, 2001; Link, Phelan, Bresnahan, Stueve, & Pescosolido, 2004; Phelan, Bromet, & Link, 1998). Because psychological disorders are more prevalent among younger cohorts, we controlled for it in all analyses. Though psychological disorder was the only medical condition controlled for specifically, we controlled for the number of medical conditions reported as it served as a measure of comorbidity (Wallace & Herzog, 1995).

Characteristics of the Respondent's Social Network

Though social networks are made up of both family and nonfamily members, this study considered only family members and any coresident nonfamily. These members provide the majority of instrumental support to an individual with ADL or IADL limitations (Messeri et al., 1993). In examining the availability of care in chapter 4, we used the following variables to break down social networks: average number of adult daughters, adult sons, brothers, sisters, living parents, and total network size, which is the summation of all relatives. We also determined the presence of a spouse and whether or not the respondent had any social network members at all.

Characteristics of the Caregiving Network

The respondent's caregiving network consisted of members of the social network previously described, other nonkin who lived in the community, and formal help. Important characteristics included the size and structure of the network. Size included the number of individuals who assisted the respondent with at least one ADL or IADL in the month prior to the survey. We divided the network into two groups: formal and informal helpers. Research indicates that the greater the number of informal helpers a person has, the fewer the hours that are provided by the primary caregiver (LaPlante et al., 2002). The number of formal helpers, however, does not impact hours of care by the primary caregiver (LaPlante et al.).

We measured the structure of the care network in a number of ways. First, we used a four-category variable to indicate whether a care network consisted of (a) a spouse only, (b) informal only (may include a spouse), (c) formal only, or (d) both formal and informal help. In some analyses, we also used a dichotomous measure indicating any formal care. The relationship of the primary caregiver to the respondent was also important and included spouse (as was previously stated, this included nonmarried partners), child, other relative, nonrelative, and formal assistant.

Characteristics of the Two Most Prevalent Primary Caregivers—Spouses and Children

The characteristics of spousal and child caregivers were important for two specific subanalyses presented in chapter 7. For spouses, we examined work status, the presence of functional limitations, and whether or not the spouse was also caring for a parent and/or dependent children. All of these may have a negative impact on a spouse's availability to care for a husband or wife who is functionally limited. We considered a number of characteristics of the respondent's children for a parallel analysis and included gender, age, marital status, work status, proximity to respondent, number of own children, and home ownership.

ANALYTIC METHODS

The HRS sampling design was multistage, stratified, and clustered (Health and Retirement Study, 2000), and therefore, we used survey sampling techniques within the Stata statistical package (Statacorp, 2003) to take the complexity of the survey design into account.

In the following, we organize the description of our analytic approach by key analytic study objectives. The first study objective was to describe the sociodemographic characteristics and social networks of individuals in late middle age who reported functional limitations and compare them to their older counterparts, as well as further describe age differences in their resultant care networks. The first objective is descriptive and is found in the first part of chapter 4 and all of chapter 5. In chapter 4, among respondents with limitations in ADLs or IADLs, we first stratified the population by age group and then calculated and compared summary statistics (means, variances) of the distribution of sociodemographic variables, casemix characteristics, and social network characteristics. Differences between age groups were tested using *t* tests. We repeated age comparisons of casemix and sociodemographic characteristics in chapter 5 for respondents who reported difficulty with at least one ADL and/or IADL as before and reported receiving at least a minimal amount of care in the month prior to the survey. For this sample, instead of examining social network characteristics, we focused on the characteristics of the care network. Again, we stratified by age and tested differences using *t* tests. Because the size and structure of the actual care network depends partly on the level of need of the individual, we used regression models to test for significant age differences in network characteristics after controlling for respondent casemix.

The second objective was to determine whether social network characteristics influenced the likelihood of receiving care, controlling for other sociodemographic characteristics, as well as respondent casemix. We describe these results in chapter 4. We examined the receipt of informal care and the receipt of formal care separately, and we examined informal care using a series of logistic regression models, the outcome of which was any receipt of informal care. Results are presented as odds ratios. The use of any formal care was rare, particularly for individuals in late middle age, allowing examination only of bivariate relationships stratified by age.

The third objective was to determine whether age-associated structural differences in helping networks influenced the amount of care received, controlling for other sociodemographic characteristics and respondent casemix. Using multivariate analysis for the third objective, we examined whether helping network characteristics (e.g., the size and composition of the network, the relation of the primary caregiver to the recipient, and/or receipt of any formal care) were associated with the amount of care received. Chapter 6 examines both total care provided and care provided solely by the primary caregiver. Chapter 7 looks further into the amount of care given by the two most prominent primary caregivers: spouses and children.

It is possible that an age difference in hours of care might be due to reporting bias. We examined this possibility in two ways. First, although the measure was considered a continuous variable, the distribution was not smooth. There was a pattern of clumping around one hour interval increases per day per month such that spikes in the distribution occurred at multiples of 30 hours. If one age group was more likely than another to show this clumping pattern, this might indicate some reporting bias. To examine this possibility, we compared the percentage of respondents in each age group who fell on a multiple of 30 and found that there was no overall difference between the groups. Just over 40% of respondents' reported hours in each age group fell on a multiple of 30.

Another possibility of reporting bias worth considering was that individuals who were older old might be more inclined to say that they had around the clock care, perhaps artificially inflating the difference in care between the young and old age groups. We examined reports of 720 hours of care or greater, which corresponds to a minimum of 24 hours of care per day over the course of the past month. Indeed, in our sample, individuals who were older old were more than twice as likely as those in late middle age to report 720 hours or more of care in the past month (10% vs. 4%, $p < .001$). However, when respondents with 720 hours or more were removed from the sample, the bivariate relationship between age and hours of care remained strong and positive. Therefore, given this and the examination of clumping, it is reasonable to believe that any age differences in hours of care found in this study are real, and not a by-product of report bias by age group.

Two transformations to hours of care were made prior to analyses. The first eliminated the most obvious outliers. Hours of care was based on a 30 day month. Therefore, a maximum of 720 (30×24) hours per month of care was allowed in the measure. This would indicate around-the-clock care from one person on average. Although it was possible for individuals to receive help from more than one individual at a time, and could therefore technically have received more than 720 hours of care in any given month, we recoded any report above 720 hours to 720. This accounted for 13 cases among individuals in late middle age (2%), 14 cases among the young old group (3%) and 64 cases among the older old group (6%).

The truncation eliminated the few instances where the help from the primary caregiver was reported as being over 24 hours per day, every day, which was possible when care by a child and his or her spouse were considered together. This caused primary caregiver hours to exceed 720 in 3 cases among individuals in late middle age (0.5%), 3 cases among the young old group (0.6%), and 14 cases among the older old group (1.3%). This was a conservative approach and, if anything, made our hypothesis (that individuals in late middle age receive fewer hours of care than the older old group) potentially more difficult to prove.

Due to the continuous nature of the dependent variable, hours of care, ordinary least squares (OLS) regression was used for these analyses. As is standard practice when studying hours of care (e.g., LaPlante et al., 2004), the second transformation was a natural log transformation of hours of care. This transformation normalized the residuals in order to better meet the underlying assumptions of OLS regression. Therefore, all analyses involving hours of care modeled log hours.

Finally, the fourth objective examined the possibility that there were not only age differences in the outcomes of interest, but that social and/or care network characteristics had a different effect on care outcomes across age groups. That is, we tested age interactions with a number of social network variables in the informal care models in chapter 4 and helping network variables in the log hours of care models in chapters 6 and 7. In order not to overload the models, these interactions were entered one-by-one, and only significant results were presented. When the number of interactions tested was greater than three or four, we used a Bonferroni adjustment to the p value to adjust for the greater likelihood of finding a significant interaction by chance alone because of multiple comparisons.

The next chapter is the first analytic chapter. We examined age differences in the likelihood of receiving care among individuals who reported difficulty performing at least one ADL or IADL. We examined the receipt of informal care and formal care separately.

Endnote

1. Twenty-four hours per day for 30 days is the equivalent of 720 hours. Some respondents reported days and hours that summed to greater than 720 hours, and so in these cases, we replaced a higher value with 720, or "24 hours per day."

Chapter 4

The Receipt of Care

There is an important distinction to be made between the availability of any care for individuals with functional limitations and receiving adequate amounts of care, measured in this study as number of hours per month. In this first analytic chapter, we examine determinants of the former, that is, whether or not individuals who reported at least one ADL and/or IADL difficulty received any help. The focus of these analyses, as throughout, was on differences in the determinants of and receipt of care by age group. Refer to figure 2.1. This chapter focused on the associations between the characteristics of individuals with functional limitations and the social network (columns 1 and 2), as well as on their association with the receipt of any community-based care. Informal and formal (paid) care were examined separately.

Past research has shown that only a small percentage of individuals aged 18 and older with functional limitations report unmet need as a result of not having a caregiver (Lima & Allen, 2001), but it is unclear whether or not this type of unmet need differs by age. At high levels of disability, it is very difficult to sustain life in the community if one does not have any assistance, and many of these individuals are institutionalized. Individuals prefer to age in place (Gitlin, 2003), and given that nursing homes have strict eligibility guidelines at least partially based on ADL functioning, there are undoubtedly many individuals with ADL difficulties left in the community, regardless of the availability of community-based care.

Here, we considered that the receipt of care by a person with reported functional difficulties depended on a number of factors. They included (a) the need for care, (b) access to care providers, and (c) preferences of care. Informal care (care provided by family and friends) and formal care (paid nonrelatives in the community) were considered separately. Given the background and theory presented earlier, we expected that individuals in late middle age with limitations in function would be less likely to receive both informal and formal care compared to their older counterparts. Through age interactions with key characteristics, we also examined whether the relationship between social network variables and the receipt of care differed by age.

Sociodemographic Characteristics of Persons With Functional Limitations

To begin, we examined the sociodemographic characteristics of persons with functional limitations in the context of age. See results in table 4.1. Forty-four percent of individuals in late middle age were male—and, as expected, there were fewer men

TABLE 4.1. Sociodemographic characteristics for individuals who report difficulty performing at least one ADL or IADL.

					Significant Difference?		
Respondent Characteristics	**All Ages (*n* = 4,000)**	**50–64 (LM) (*n* = 1,234)**	**65–74 (YO) (*n* = 1,069)**	**75+ (OO) (*n* = 1,697)**	**LM vs. YO**	**LM vs. OO**	**YO vs. OO**
	% (*SE*)	% (*SE*)	% (*SE*)	% (*SE*)			
Male	39.0% (0.8%)	44.1% (1.3%)	39.8% (1.5%)	34.1% (1.1%)	*	***	**
Race/Ethnicity							
Non-Hispanic White	75.9% (1.8%)	70.4% (2.2%)	73.3% (2.4%)	82.5% (1.9%)		***	***
Non-Hispanic Black	13.6% (1.0%)	16.3% (1.3%)	14.5% (1.5%)	10.5% (1.4%)		***	*
Hispanic	8.4% (1.6%)	10.6% (2.1%)	10.0% (2.1%)	5.4% (1.4%)		**	**
Other	2.1% (0.5%)	2.7% (0.7%)	2.2% (0.7%)	1.6% (0.5%)			
Education							
Less than high school	40.6% (1.4%)	34.8% (2.3%)	42.2% (1.9%)	44.7% (1.6%)	**	***	
High school	32.8% (1.0%)	35.5% (2.2%)	32.1% (1.7%)	30.9% (1.0%)		*	
More than high school	26.6% (1.1%)	29.8% (1.8%)	25.8% (2.0%)	24.4% (1.2%)		*	
Marital Status							
Married/ partnered	52.3% (1.1%)	64.4% (1.6%)	56.4% (2.3%)	39.0% (1.3%)	**	***	***
Divorced/ separated	13.0% (0.7%)	20.9% (1.3%)	13.4% (1.5%)	5.8% (0.8%)	***	***	***

(*continued on next page*)

TABLE 4.1. *(continued)*

Respondent Characteristics	All Ages (n = 4,000)	50–64 (LM) (n = 1,234)	65–74 (YO) (n = 1,069)	75+ (OO) (n = 1,697)	Significant Difference? LM vs. YO	LM vs. OO	YO vs. OO
Marital Status							
Widowed	30.4% (0.9%)	8.8% (0.8%)	25.9% (1.5%)	52.4% (1.3%)	***	***	***
Never married	4.3% (0.5%)	5.9% (1.1%)	4.3% (0.7%)	2.9% (0.3%)		**	
Insurance[a]							
Medicare (1/0)	73.5% (1.0%)	29.7% (1.6%)	95.8% (0.8%)	98.0% (0.4%)	***	***	**
Medicaid (1/0)	16.6% (1.2%)	17.0% (1.4%)	19.6% (1.9%)	14.2% (1.4%)			**
Private (1/0)	35.9% (1.3%)	51.1% (1.8%)	29.7% (1.7%)	26.3% (1.6%)	***	***	
No insurance (1/0)	4.2% (0.5%)	11.1% (1.2%)	0.8% (0.2%)	0.3% (0.1%)	***	***	
Currently Working for Pay	15.8% (0.8%)	32.9% (1.7%)	11.9% (1.2%)	3.3% (0.5%)	***	***	***
Household Income[b]							
Quintile 1	36.5% (1.3%)	33.0% (2.3%)	36.6% (2.1%)	39.4% (1.4%)		**	
Quintile 2	24.5% (0.8%)	16.0% (1.2%)	27.0% (1.9%)	30.5% (1.2%)	***	***	
Quintile 3	17.0% (0.8%)	17.8% (1.7%)	17.2% (1.4%)	16.2% (0.9%)			
Quintile 4	12.4% (0.8%)	17.4% (1.5%)	11.3% (0.9%)	8.7% (0.8%)	***	***	**
Quintile 5	9.6% (0.6%)	15.9% (1.5%)	7.9% (1.0%)	5.1% (0.5%)	***	***	*

Note. LM = late middle age; YO = young old; OO = older old.

[a]Insurance categories are not mutually exclusive.

[b]Household income for those 50+ in general population was divided into five equal groups. This shows the percent for this subpopulation within each quintile.

$*p < .05$. $**p < .01$. $***p < .001$.

in older groups (39.8% among the young old group and 34.1% among the older old group), likely because of the lower life expectancies of males (Hobbs & Stoops, 2002).

Comparisons of other demographic characteristics, such as race/ethnicity, marital history, and education, reflected the timing of the major demographic transitions in the lives of these three groups that took place in the latter half of the 20th century (i.e., cohort differences). Specifically, individuals in late middle age were similar in racial and ethnic composition to those in the young old group, but were more ethnically diverse than the older old group. They consisted of 60% more Blacks (16.3% vs. 10.5%, $p < .001$) and nearly twice as many Hispanics (10.6% vs. 5.4%, $p < .01$) than the older old group. Late-middle-aged adults were less likely than either group to have less than a high school education (34.8% vs. 42.2% and 44.7%). They were also more likely than the older old group to have furthered their education beyond high school (29.8% vs. 24.3%, $p < .05$), but they did not differ from the young old group in that respect.

The likelihood of being currently married decreased significantly with age, from 64.4% among individuals in late middle age to 39.0% among individuals who were older old ($p < .001$), as did the likelihood of being divorced. Twenty-one percent (20.9%) of late-middle-aged adults were divorced at the time of the survey, compared with 13.4% among the young old group ($p < .001$) and 6% among the older old group ($p < .001$). Conversely, more than half of the older old group were widowed (52.4%) compared with only 26% of the young old group ($p < .001$) and 9% of the late-middle-aged group ($p < .\ 001$). Individuals in late middle age were twice as likely as older old adults to have never married (5.9% vs. 2.9%, $p < .01$), although they did not differ significantly from young old adults in this regard.

Because of Medicare, virtually all adults aged 65 and older had at least some insurance, but 11% of those under 65 were uninsured at the time of the survey ($p < .001$). Medicaid rates were similar across groups, and private health insurance was more common among the late-middle-aged group compared with older groups. And, while close to one-third of those in late middle age were still working at the time of the survey (33%), only 12% ($p < .001$) of those in the young old group and 3% ($p < .001$) of the older old group were doing so.

As mentioned in chapter 3, household income for the general population 50 and older in the HRS was divided into quintiles. As table 4.1 demonstrates, individuals who reported limitations in function had lower incomes, on average, than the general population, with approximately 60% of respondents falling into the bottom two quintiles (see first column). Among those with functional limitations, household income decreased with age such that approximately 49% of late-middle-aged adults, 64% of young old adults, and 70% of older old adults fell within the bottom two quintiles.

DID THEIR HEALTH AND FUNCTIONING DIFFER BY AGE?

When examining age differences in the receipt of care, it was important to demonstrate that any age difference found was not due simply to differences in the need for care. To do this, we controlled for respondent casemix. Table 4.2 provides frequencies of respondent casemix by age.

Overall, as one might expect, older old adults appeared to be more infirm than younger adults. Respondents did not differ by age in the number of ADL difficulties reported (1.55 to 1.61, range 0–6), although IADL difficulty increased with age

TABLE 4.2. Respondent casemix for individuals who report difficulty performing at least one ADL or IADL.

Respondent Characteristics	All Ages (*n* = 4,000)	50–64 (LM) (*n* = 1,234)	65–74 (YO) (*n* = 1,069)	75+ (OO) (*n* = 1,697)	Significant Difference? LM vs. YO	LM vs. OO	YO vs. OO
Number of ADL Difficulties (*M*, *SE*)	1.59, .03	1.61, .06	1.55, .04	1.61, .04			
Number of IADL Difficulties (*M*, *SE*)	1.19, .03	0.97, .04	1.03, .05	1.50, .05		***	***
Number of Hospitalizations in Past 2 Years (*M*, *SE*)	5.26, .35	4.24, .34	5.48, .42	6.01, .66	*	*	
Number of Bed Days in Past Month (*M*, *SE*)	2.63, .15	3.17, .27	2.60, .28	2.17, .18		**	
	% (*SE*)	% (*SE*)	% (*SE*)	% (*SE*)			
Easily Fatigued/Exhausted in Past 2 Weeks	42.8% (0.8%)	48.3% (1.6%)	38.7% (1.3%)	40.4% (1.4%)	***	***	
General Health							
Excellent	2.7% (0.3%)	2.9% (0.6%)	2.1% (0.4%)	3.0% (0.5%)			
Very good	10.5% (0.6%)	9.0% (1.0%)	10.3% (1.1%)	11.8% (1.0%)			
Good	25.7% (0.9%)	22.9% (1.6%)	27.1% (1.6%)	27.2% (1.4%)		*	
Fair	33.3% (0.9%)	34.2% (1.7%)	32.9% (1.8%)	32.8% (1.2%)			
Poor	27.8% (1.0%)	30.9% (1.6%)	27.6% (1.8%)	25.3% (1.37%)		*	
Wheelchair Use	7.3% (0.5%)	5.9% (1.0%)	6.7% (0.8%)	8.9% (0.8%)		*	
Psychological Disorder	26.9% (1.0%)	36.2% (1.7%)	24.6% (1.6%)	20.2% (1.0%)	***	***	*
Cognitive Impairment	10.3% (0.6%)	3.6% (0.5%)	9.2% (1.2%)	17.0% (1.0%)	***	***	***

(*continued on next page*)

Table 4.2. *(continued)*

Respondent Characteristics	All Ages (n = 4,000)	50–64 (LM) (n = 1,234)	65–74 (YO) (n = 1,069)	75+ (OO) (n = 1,697)	Significant Difference? LM vs. YO	LM vs. OO	YO vs. OO
Pain	59.7% (0.9%)	71.5% (1.6%)	58.5% (1.6%)	50.0% (1.2%)	***	***	***
Number of Medical Conditions (*M*, *SE*)	2.72, 0.30	2.54, 0.05	2.82, 0.05	2.80, 0.0	***	**	
Body Mass Index							
Underweight (BMI < 18.5)	3.9% (0.4%)	1.3% (0.4%)	3.7% (0.8%)	6.2% (0.7%)	*	***	*
Normal/obese	90.7% (0.5%)	88.7% (1.2%)	90.7% (1.0%)	92.6% (0.7%)		*	
Morbidly obese (BMI > 40)	5.4% (0.4%)	9.9% (1.18%)	5.6% (0.7%)	1.3% (0.3%)	**	***	***

Note. LM = late middle age; YO = young old; OO = older old.
*$p < .05$. **$p < .01$. ***$p < .001$.

(from an average of 0.97 among those in late middle age to 1.50 among the older old group, $p < .001$).

Individuals in late middle age spent fewer nights in the hospital in the 2 years prior to the survey than either the young old or older old group ($p < .01$), but they spent more days in bed in the month prior to the survey compared with the older old group ($p < .01$). They were more likely to be easily fatigued or exhausted (48.3%) compared with those who were young old (38.7%) or older old (40.4%, $p < .001$).

Over one-quarter of each age group considered their health to be poor. Less than 10% of respondents reported the use of a wheelchair, but this increased from 6% among individuals in late middle age to 9% among those who were older old ($p < .05$). Over one-third of late-middle-aged individuals (36.2%) reported a psychological disorder compared with 25% of the young old group ($p < .001$) and 20% of the older old group ($p < .001$). Conversely, cognitive impairment increased significantly with age from 4% to 9% to 17% across the three age groups ($p < .001$). The report of pain decreased significantly by age ($p < .001$).

Finally, while the vast majority of respondents had a body mass index ranging from normal to obese (91% of total sample), late-middle-aged adults who did not fall within that range were almost entirely morbidly obese, while those in the older old group who did not fall within that range were almost entirely underweight. Among those who were young old, those who did not fall within the normal/obese range were more evenly divided, such that 4% were underweight and 6% were morbidly obese.

Social Network Characteristics

Table 4.3 presents characteristics of the respondents' familial social networks. Though information on nonrelatives was

TABLE 4.3. Social network characteristics for individuals who report difficulty performing at least one ADL or IADL.

					Significant Difference?		
	All Ages (n = 4,000)	**50–64 (LM) (n = 1,234)**	**65–74 (YO) (n = 1,069)**	**75+ (OO) (n = 1,697)**	**LM vs. YO**	**LM vs. OO**	**YO vs. OO**
Total Social Network[a] (*M*, *SE*)	5.39, 0.11	7.37, 0.15	5.24, 0.13	3.72, 0.08	***	***	***
Average Number of	**(*M*, *SE*)**	**(*M*, *SE*)**	**(*M*, *SE*)**	**(*M*, *SE*)**			
Adult daughters	1.40, 0.03	1.31, 0.04	1.58, 0.05	1.35, 0.03	***		***
Adult sons	1.48, 0.03	1.41, 0.04	1.70, 0.04	1.38, 0.04	***		***
Sisters	1.34, 0.03	1.69, 0.06	1.44, 0.05	0.95, 0.03	***	***	***
Brothers	1.12, 0.03	1.56, 0.06	1.17, 0.04	0.69, 0.02	***	***	***
Parents	0.31, 0.02	0.73, 0.03	0.18, 0.01	0.01, 0.00	***	***	***
Has Any	**% (*SE*)**	**% (*SE*)**	**% (*SE*)**	**% (*SE*)**			
Daughter	78.2% (0.9%)	76.0% (1.6%)	79.9% (1.4%)	79.1% (1.0%)			
Son	70.4% (0.7%)	69.7% (1.8%)	76.6% (1.2%)	67.0% (1.1%)	**		***
Sister	63.7% (1.0%)	73.3% (1.6%)	67.6% (2.0%)	52.8% (1.3%)	*	***	***
Brother	57.5% (0.9%)	71.6% (1.6%)	62.0% (1.5%)	42.4% (1.3%)	***	***	***
Parent/-in-law	21.8% (1.1%)	48.7% (1.9%)	16.2% (1.6%)	1.7% (0.3%)	***	***	***
Has no social network member	2.2% (0.3%)	1.0% (0.6%)	1.6% (0.5%)	3.7% (0.4%)		***	**

Note. LM = late middle age; YO = young old; OO = older old.
[a]Total social network = number of household members, living siblings, children, and parents/-in-law.
*$p < .05$. **$p < .01$. ***$p < .001$.

not available, family members are more likely than friends to provide the type of instrumental support that was considered in this study.

Late-middle-aged adults had the largest overall social networks, compared with either those who were young old or older old when we considered spouses, children, siblings, and parents. On average, they had over seven network members (7.4), while those who were young old had 5.2 ($p < .001$), and those who were older old had 3.7 ($p < .001$). This was primarily because they had more living brothers, sisters, and parents than did their older counterparts ($p < .001$). Young old adults, however, had significantly more adult children (both sons and daughters) than either late-middle-aged ($p < .001$) or older old adults ($p < .001$) who did not differ from one another. This reflects the timing of the baby boom, when an increase in fertility rates followed World War II.

In the context of caregiving, perhaps the number of family members is not as important as the presence of particular members. Table 4.1 reports that individuals in late middle age were the most likely to have a spouse compared with either the young old or the older old group. As table 4.3 indicates, the presence of other family members also differed by age. All age groups were equally likely to have at least one daughter (78.2% overall), but young old adults were more likely than both late-middle-aged and older old adults to report having at least one son. As one might expect, the likelihood of having at least one living brother, sister, or parent (separately) decreased significantly with age. And while the vast majority of each age group had at least one living family member, the older old group was significantly more likely than either younger group to be without any social network member ($p < .01$).

A First Look at the Relationship Between Receipt of Help and Age

Partly likely because of these differences in casemix, sociodemographic, and social network characteristics, figure 4.1 demonstrates that at the bivariate level, younger respondents were significantly less likely than their older old counterparts to report receiving help with ADLs and/or IADLs. Only 48% of late-middle-aged respondents and 50% of the young old respondents reported receiving any help, compared with 63% of older old respondents ($p < .001$). Those who were young old did not differ significantly from late-middle-aged respondents in this regard.

When considering informal care and formal care separately, the results were similar for the receipt of informal care such that

FIGURE 4.1. Bivariate relationship between age and receipt of care.

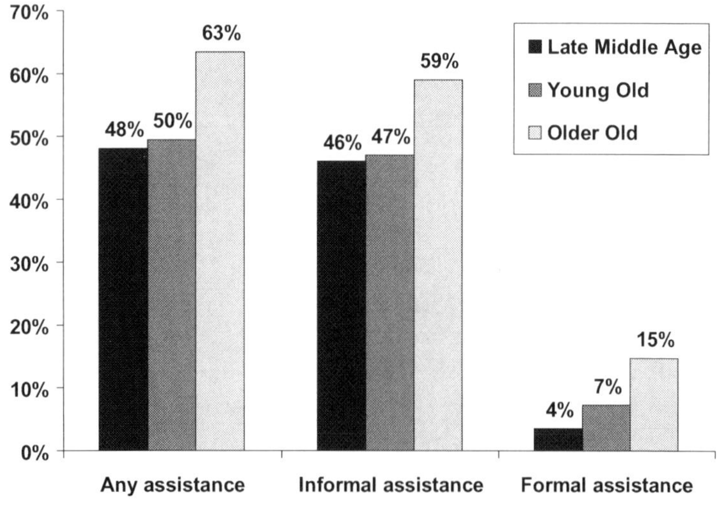

late-middle-aged and young old individuals were less likely to receive care compared with the older old group, although they did not differ from one another. For the receipt of formal care, the likelihood of receiving care increased significantly with each age, such that those who were young old were more likely to receive formal care than those in late middle age while the older old group was more likely than either group to do so.

Multivariate Results of Receipt of Informal Care

We just saw that on the bivariate level, late-middle-aged and young old adults were less likely to receive any informal care with ADL or IADL activities, even though the presence of social network members would suggest that there were more, not fewer, potential caregivers to call upon. Does this lower receipt of care reflect simply a lower need for care on the part of the younger age groups? No—even after controlling for casemix, sociodemographic characteristics, and social network characteristics, late-middle-aged adults were 28% less likely than their older old counterparts to receive informal care ($p < .05$; odds ratio [OR] = .72; see table 4.4). Those who were young old were 37% less likely than the older old group to do so ($p = .001$; OR = .63).

We ran a series of regressions that included the various social network characteristics presented in table 4.3. Only two social network variables were significant. Presence of an adult daughter[1] was positively associated with receiving informal care, while the absence of any family social network member was negatively associated with receiving informal care when entered separately. When these two variables were entered together, as shown in table 4.4, both remained statistically significant.

TABLE 4.4. Logistic regression of the receipt of informal care for individuals who report difficulty performing at least one ADL or IADL.

	OR (95% CI)
Constant	0.56 (0.28, 1.11)
Age (ref: 75+)	
50–64	0.72 (0.54, 0.95)*
65–74	0.63 (0.48, 0.81)**
Currently Working	0.46 (0.34, 0.64)***
Male	0.85 (0.64, 1.13)
Lives Alone	0.27 (0.19, 0.38)***
Marital Status (ref: married/partnered)	
Divorced/separated	0.70 (0.47, 1.05)
Widowed	0.72 (0.53, 0.97)*
Never married	0.69 (0.39, 1.21)
Education (ref: high school)	
Less than high school	1.09 (0.85, 1.41)
More than high school	0.86 (0.65, 1.13)
Race/Ethnicity (ref: non-Hispanic White)	
Black	1.09 (0.83, 1.44)
Hispanic	0.79 (0.51, 1.24)
Other	0.93 (0.49, 1.75)
Medicaid	0.93 (0.68, 1.27)
Household Income (ref: Quintile 1)	
Quintile 2	0.90 (0.70, 1.16)
Quintile 3	0.61 (0.42, 0.90)*
Quintile 4	0.73 (0.51, 1.04)
Quintile 5	0.87 (0.55, 1.37)
Has Daughter	1.32 (1.03, 1.69)*
Has No Social Network Member	0.51 (0.26, 0.97)*
N	3845
F(nDF, dDF)	(33, 20) = 15.58
prob. > *F*	0.000

Note. All models control for respondent casemix (number of ADL difficulties, number of IADL difficulties, number of nights in hospital, fatigue, number of days in bed, wheelchair use, general health, presence of a psychological disorder, pain, number of medical conditions, and body mass index). OR = odds ratio; CI = confidence interval.
**p* < .05. ***p* < .01. ****p* < .001.

Respondents who had an adult daughter in their network were 32% more likely to receive informal care compared with those without an adult daughter ($p < .05$). Having no one in one's network reduced one's likelihood of receiving care by half (OR = 0.51, $p < .05$). Interestingly, the number of total social network members was not significantly associated with the receipt of care (not shown).

We next tested a number of interactions. Perhaps, for instance, the number of social network members is not associated with the receipt of care for the older old group but it is for the late-middle-aged group. To consider this and other possibilities, we tested age interactions with marital status and various social network characteristics.

We expected current marital status to be the sociodemographic characteristic with the most potential to interact with age as it affects the receipt of care. Widowhood was more common among those who were older old, and widowhood earlier in life may evoke strong emotions that make family and friends around the widow/widower in need of assistance more likely to reach out. Or perhaps this uncommon event among late-middle-aged couples may evoke a feeling of loneliness on the part of the widow/widower in need prompting him or her to reject offers of assistance. Finally, divorce rates have been high since the 1970s. Perhaps the negative effect of divorce on social support (Pezzin & Schone, 1999) among elders was not so pronounced among younger cohorts for whom divorce was more common.

We also tested interactions with age for the overall number in the social network, whether or not there was any social network member, the presence of adult daughters, and the presence of sisters. Given the possibility that the social networks of those in late middle age were younger in general than the older old group and that these members may have had more competing demands than social network members of the older old group, it was possible that having more network members was important for late-middle-aged adults but not for those who were older old. For the older old group, just having a social network member may have sufficed. Finally, given the general importance of females as caregivers (Stone et al., 1987), we tested two gendered social network interactions. Daughters are known to be important caregivers to elderly parents, but it is unclear whether or not they play as big a role to parents who are younger. In addition, in the absence of others, sisters may play important roles in the caregiving networks of those in late middle age.

In total, we formally tested five interactions, and each was entered into the model separately. Because the number of tests alone increased the likelihood of finding a significant interaction just by chance, we used a Bonferroni adjustment to determine the p value that would account for multiple comparisons. Starting with a p value of .05 and adjusting for five comparisons, we considered only a p value of .01 or lower to be significant (.05/5).

Only the interaction between age and marital status showed a significant result with a p value lower than .01 and only for divorced young old adults versus older old adults. Results are displayed in table 4.5. Specifically, young old adults who were divorced were 88% less likely than older old adults who were divorced to receive any informal care (0.21). Derivation of the adjusted odds ratio can be found in appendix A. In results not shown, they were also less likely than late-middle-aged adults to do so, although the p value reached only $p < .03$.

Table 4.5. Logistic regression model including age/marital status interaction for individuals who report difficulty performing at least one ADL or IADL.

	OR (95% CI)
Constant	0.24 (.68, 1.27)*
Age (ref: 75+)	
50–64	0.82 (0.59, 1.13)
65–74	0.76 (0.56, 1.04)
Marital Status (ref: married/partnered)	
Divorced/separated	1.17 (0.67, 2.04)
Widowed	0.89 (0.62, 1.30)
Never married	0.81 (0.29, 2.24)
Age × Marital Status (ref: married older old)	
50–64 × Divorced/separated	0.71 (0.36, 1.42)
50–64 × Widowed	0.44 (0.2, 0.94)
50–64 × Never married	0.81 (0.16, 4.04)
65–74 × Divorced/separated	0.28 (0.12, 0.63)*
65–74 × Widowed	0.82 (0.5, 1.35)
65–74 × Never married	0.91 (0.25, 3.24)
N	3,845
***F*(*nDF*, *dDF*)**	(39, 14) = 17.85
prob. > *F*	0.000

Note. Model also controls for the sociodemographic, casemix, and social network characteristics included in table 4.4. OR = odds ratio, CI = confidence interval.
$^*p < .01$.

Description of the Receipt of Formal Care by Age

Setting aside informal care for the moment, we then turned our attention to formal care. An extensive examination of the receipt of formal care was difficult because very few people in late middle age received any formal care. Only 4% of persons aged 50–64 with functional difficulty reported having any type of formal care in the month prior to the survey. This was compared with 7% of the young old group ($p < .01$) and 15% of the older old group ($p < .001$). Because access to disability services is often age based (Allen & Mor, 1997), which limits the availability of services to late-middle-aged persons and also may skew their perceptions about the acceptability of using formal care at their age, we suspected that the factors that influenced the receipt of formal care differed by age. Therefore, presenting a main effects model similar to the informal care models just described would be misleading. However, given the small sample size, particularly among late-middle-aged adults, a stratified multivariate analysis was not possible. For that reason, we present only a limited descriptive look at the receipt of formal care.

We present bivariate relationships between sociodemographic characteristics and formal care, as well as between social network characteristics and formal care, in a series of bar charts. Each age group was examined separately. Tables of percentages and standard errors for the figures are available in appendix B. Figures 4.2a–c present the bivariate relationships for those in late middle age. Figures 4.3a–c and 4.4a–c present them for the young old and older old groups, respectively. Though casemix was not controlled, given the large difference in the percentage that received any formal care by age, it is unlikely that casemix accounted for all of the difference.

At first glance, figure 4.2a paints a clear picture of formal care users among those in late middle age. They were likely to be poor, widowed, and on Medicaid. They lacked a high school degree and were not working at the time of the study. Recall from figure 4.1 that, overall, only 4% of those in late middle age received any formal care. Those who were widowed, however, were more than 12 times as likely as those who were currently married to receive any formal care (16.1% vs. 1.3%, $p < .001$). Though

FIGURE 4.2A. Bivariate relationship between the receipt of any formal help and select sociodemographic characteristics for individuals who report difficulty performing at least one ADL or IADL—late-middle-aged adults.

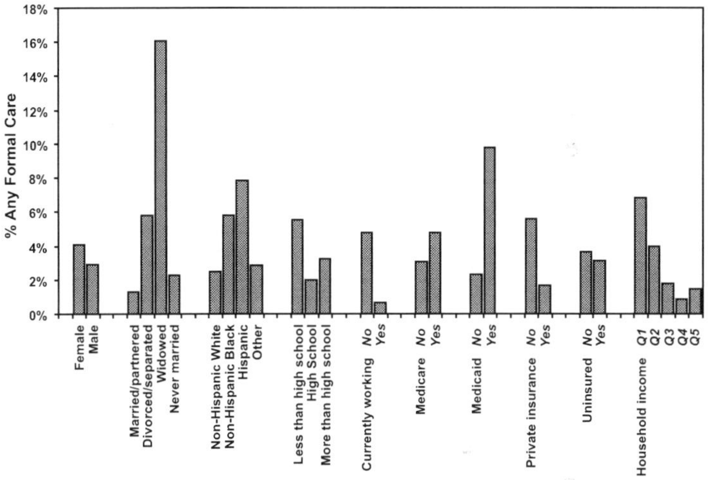

less dramatic, those who were divorced were also more likely to receive formal care than those who were currently married ($p < .05$). Those with less than a high school degree and those not currently working were more likely than those with higher education or current workers to receive formal care. This is likely related to the fact that those on Medicaid and those with the lowest income levels were more likely to receive formal care than their counterparts. These results suggest that formal care was accessible primarily through the Medicaid program, and people may have had to spend down their assets in order to receive formal care. Clearly, being in the highest income bracket did not suggest that individuals were able to purchase formal care.

FIGURE 4.2B. Bivariate relationship between the receipt of any formal help and select social network characteristics for individuals who report difficulty performing at least one ADL or IADL—late-middle-aged adults.

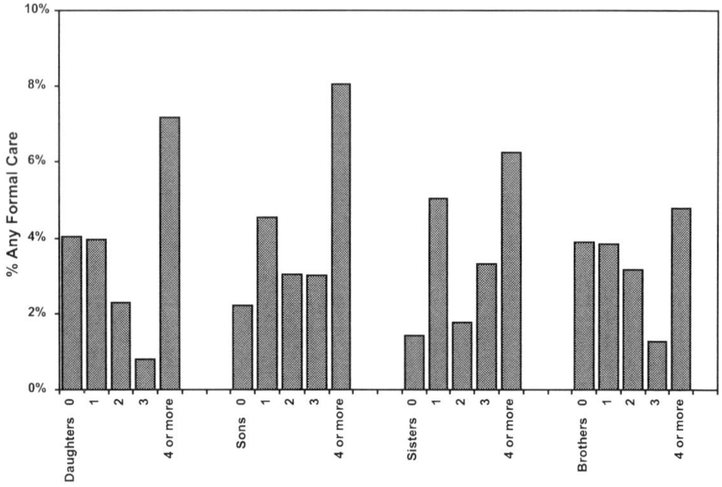

Figures 4.2b–c present social network characteristics and the receipt of formal care among late-middle-aged adults. Unlike sociodemographic characteristics, social network characteristics did not appear to play a large role in the receipt of formal care for this age group. The only characteristic that significantly affected the likelihood of receiving formal care for those in late middle age was the presence of a sister. Individuals with at least one sister were significantly more likely to receive formal care than individuals without a sister. In this instance, the sister was likely middle-aged herself, a common age when women care for elderly parents. It is conceivable that having a sister was a source of information to those in late middle age with difficulty in function. Perhaps these women were

FIGURE 4.2C. Bivariate relationship between the receipt of any formal help and more social network characteristics for individuals who report difficulty performing at least one ADL or IADL—late-middle-aged adults.

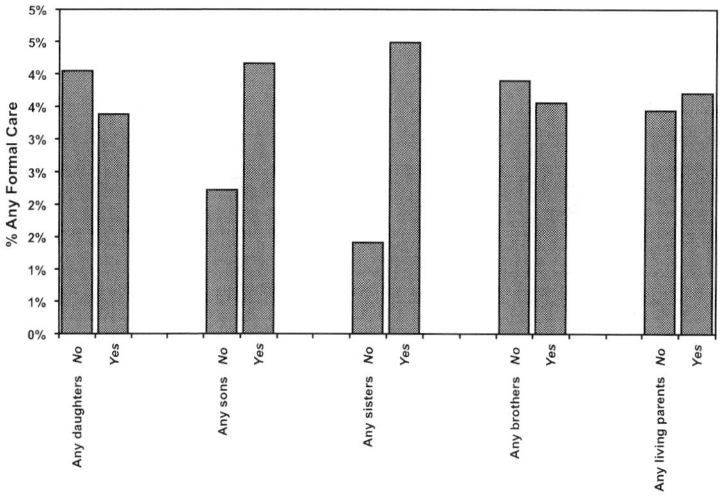

able to inform their sibling about the possibility of formal care because they had gone through the experience of obtaining it for their parents.

While none reach statistical significance, perhaps due to restrictions in sample size,[2] the graph suggests that those in late middle age with 4 or more daughters or 4 or more sons may have been more likely to receive formal care compared with those with fewer children. Though formal care may have been too expensive for small numbers of children to pay for, perhaps children pooled their money to purchase formal care for a parent when there were enough children in the family to make this feasible. Though less pronounced, this pattern was also visible for siblings of the respondent.

FIGURE 4.3A. Bivariate relationship between the receipt of any formal help and select sociodemographic characteristics for individuals who report difficulty performing at least one ADL or IADL—young old adults.

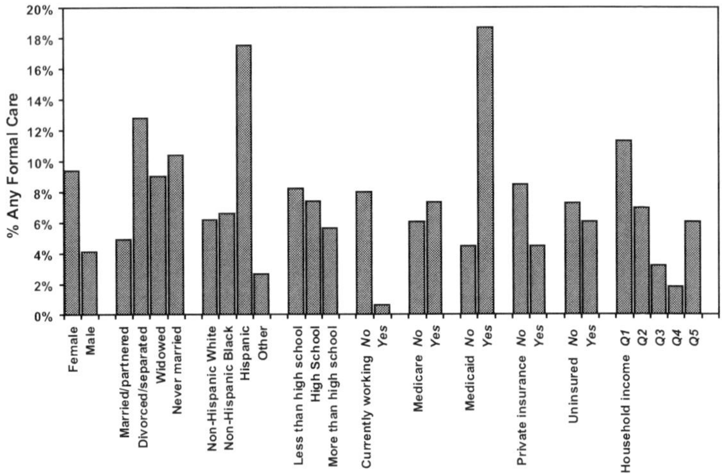

A somewhat different pattern emerged for the young old group. Figure 4.3a presents the receipt of formal care by sociodemographic characteristics. Keep in mind that twice as many young old as late-middle-aged adults received formal care (7.4% vs. 3.6%). Unlike those in late middle age, there were no significant differences in the receipt of formal care by marital status for those who were young old. Rather, women were twice as likely as men to receive some formal care (9.3% vs. 4.1%, $p < .001$). Hispanics were more likely than other race/ethnicities to do so. As was also the case for late-middle-aged adults, however, those with little income and those on Medicaid were more likely than their counterparts to receive formal care. It appears that those in the highest income bracket may have been in a position to pay for formal services. However, the percentage

FIGURE 4.3B. Bivariate relationship between the receipt of any formal help and select social network characteristics for individuals who report difficulty performing at least one ADL or IADL—young old adults.

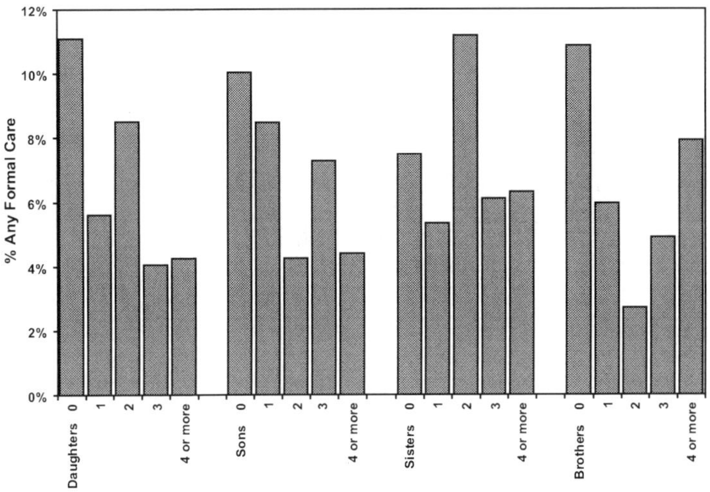

who received formal care did not differ significantly from those in the next lower quintile, although again, this may be a result of limited power.

Unlike those in late middle age, it appears that in the absence of adequate informal care, those who were young old were able to compensate with formal care. Figures 4.3b–c indicate that individuals with no sons or daughters were more likely to have formal care than those with one or more of those family members. Interestingly, however, the strong benefit of having a sister found among late-middle-aged adults was not found for this age group.

Finally, figures 4.4a–c examine the receipt of formal care among the older old group. With this third set of figures, a third

FIGURE 4.3C. Bivariate relationship between the receipt of any formal help and more social network characteristics for individuals who report difficulty performing at least one ADL or IADL—young old adults.

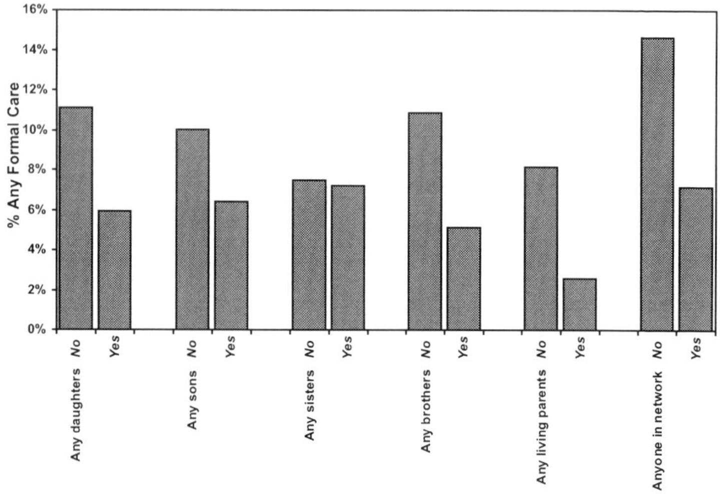

pattern emerged. Fifteen percent of those who were older old received at least some formal care (review figure 4.1). This was four times as many as the late-middle-aged group and twice and many as the young old group who did so. Females were almost twice as likely as males to receive formal care ($p < .001$). See figure 4.4a. This is likely related to the fact that those who were currently married were significantly less likely than those who were not to receive formal care, and at older ages women are more likely than men to be widowed. Hispanics were more likely than non-Hispanic Whites to receive formal care. Here, as in the other age groups, Medicaid appeared to be a driving force, such that those with Medicaid and those with

FIGURE 4.4A. Bivariate relationship between the receipt of any formal help and select sociodemographic characteristics for individuals who report difficulty performing at least one ADL or IADL—older old adults.

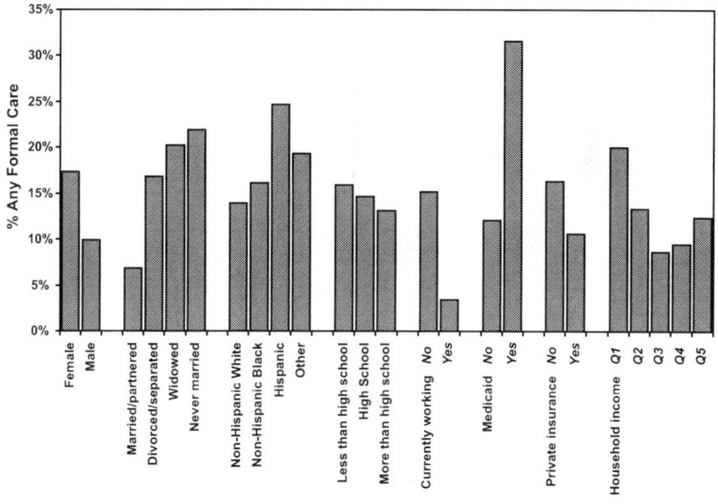

low incomes were more likely to have formal care than their counterparts.

Figure 4.4b does not show a clear pattern in terms of number of children and siblings, but figure 4.4c demonstrates that the older old group, like the young old group, were likely able to compensate somewhat for a lack of any social network member using formal care. In the absence of any social network member to provide informal care, it is difficult to sustain life in the community if one has difficulty with ADLs or IADLs without some form of formal assistance.

FIGURE 4.4B. Bivariate relationship between the receipt of any formal help and select social network characteristics for individuals who report difficulty performing at least one ADL or IADL—older old adults.

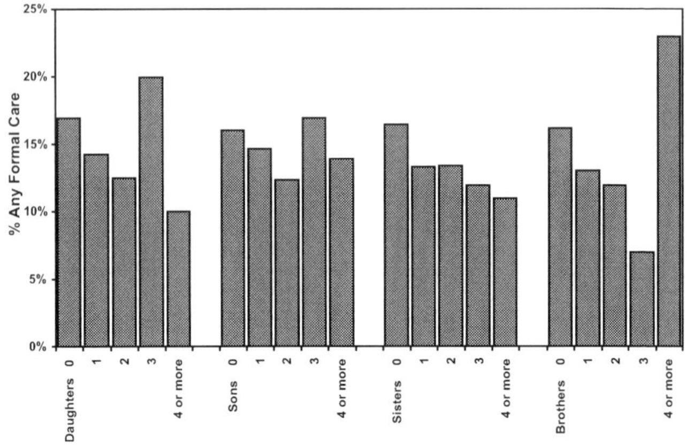

FIGURE 4.4C. Bivariate relationship between the receipt of any formal help and more social network characteristics for individuals who report difficulty performing at least one ADL or IADL—older old adults.

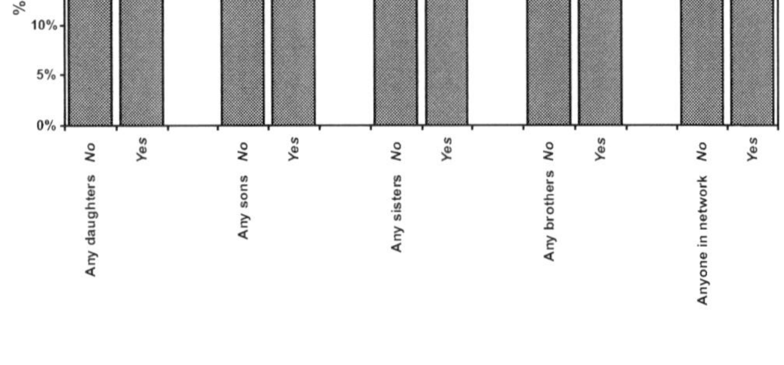

Discussion

This first set of analyses has revealed some important information about the receipt of care among persons in late middle age, information that up until now had not been confirmed. By and large, we found support for a number of hypotheses. Even after controlling for casemix, sociodemographic characteristics, and social network characteristics, both the late-middle-aged and young old groups were less likely to receive care than their older old counterparts. There are many possible explanations for these differences. For example, they could be due to differences in the supply of help when help is desired, or to differences in the demand for help given a particular level of objective need.

The first difference would suggest that the shift in demographic characteristics that has occurred over the past century has resulted in higher levels of unmet need, requiring an active effort on the part of policy makers to work toward eliminating this shortfall through various programs. It would suggest that this shortfall in informal care resources in late middle age will carry over into the older population as the population ages and may put further strain on an already strained long-term care system.

However, if the age differences are due to a decrease in the level of demand for informal assistance, then reasons for this decrease in demand would warrant further study. Even when persons in late middle age might benefit from informal help, it is possible that they may not want to lose independence or burden family members with their care.

Though only a descriptive look at the use of formal care was possible, the results are telling. That the older old group used formal services at a rate four times that of the late-middle-aged group suggests that there was a difference in accessibility between these two age groups. This difference is made that much worse when one considers that younger age groups were also less likely to receive informal care. The perception of the use of formal care among adults in late middle age should also be considered a potential barrier to its use, as should financial constraints. While these results are purely descriptive, they do suggest that adults in late middle age had limited opportunity for, and possibly awareness of, formal care services.

Endnotes

1. Number of adult daughters can be used in place of presence of an adult daughter, as both showed similar results.
2. Using NQuery Advisor, Version 5.0, power analysis software (see Elashoff, 2002), we tested how much power we had to detect a significant difference in the percentage who had formal care for late middle-aged adults with 4 or more daughters versus those with fewer than 4 daughters. Given a mean of .033 use of formal care for those with fewer than 4 daughters (n = 1,141) and a mean of .072 for those with 4 or more daughters (n = 93), a 2-group t test with a 0.05 two-sided significance level has only 26% power to detect the difference between the two groups.

Chapter 5

Care Networks

For the remainder of the study, we considered only respondents who received at least a minimum of care in the month prior to the survey. In this chapter, we discuss how we examined age differences in the types of caregivers likely to make up the care network. We expected that both the characteristics of the individual in need, as well as the characteristics of the care networks, affected the amount of care that an individual receives, controlling for casemix. Therefore, before examining hours of care, we took a descriptive look at age differences in the network characteristics themselves. We expected that the composition of the actual care network, including the relationship of the members to the recipient, as well as the combination of formal and informal services, would differ by age group. Specifically, we expected to find that compared with their older counterparts, individuals in late middle age would (a) have fewer adult children in their care networks, (b) be more likely to be receiving help from a spouse, (c) be more likely to be receiving help from informal nonkin, (d) be less likely to be receiving formal care, and (e) be less likely to have secondary caregivers (i.e., more than one caregiver). Differences here would highlight the life course concept that the timing of a transition has important consequences on the outcome (George, 2002). Specifically, most hypothesized differences reflect the differing life stages the respondents and their support networks were in at the time of their need for help.

Of the 4,000 individuals with functional limitations in the previous chapter, 2,259 (56.5%) received help in the past month performing at least one ADL or IADL task. Table 5.1 presents the sociodemographic characteristics of individuals aged 50 and older who reported receiving help with at least one ADL or IADL due to a health or memory problem. We compared these characteristics across the three age groups.

Age differences were similar to those presented in the previous chapter. Individuals in late middle age differed significantly from those who were older old in almost every respect, while those who were young old shared some characteristics with late-middle-aged adults, some with older old adults, and had some uniquely their own.

Specifically, gender and race/ethnicity distributions were similar between the late-middle-aged and the young old groups, but both of these age groups differed significantly from the older old group. Compared with those who were older old, the younger groups were composed of more males and minorities. Individuals in late middle age were more educated than either the young old or the older old groups who did not differ from one another. While 40% of those in late middle age had less than a high school education, 47% of the young old group ($p < .05$) and 49% of the older old group did so ($p < .01$).

Table 5.1. Sociodemographic characteristics by age group for individuals who receive help with at least one ADL or IADL.

Respondent Characteristics	All Ages (*n* = 2,559)	50–64 (LM) (*n* = 612)	65–74 (YO) (*n* = 540)	75+ (OO) (*n* = 1,107)	Significant Difference? LM vs. YO	LM vs. OO	YO vs. OO
	% (*SE*)	% (*SE*)	% (*SE*)	% (*SE*)			
Male	37.2% (2.0%)	41.0% (2.4%)	39.4% (2.10%)	33.6% (1.3%)		*	*
Race/Ethnicity							
Non-Hispanic White	73.6% (2.0%)	66.9% (2.5%)	69.4% (2.8%)	80.1% (2.1%)		***	***
Non-Hispanic Black	15.3% (1.5%)	18.5% (2.2%)	17.0% (2.2%)	12.2% (1.7%)		**	*
Hispanic	9.1% (1.9%)	12.0% (2.6%)	11.3% (2.3%)	6.1% (1.7%)		**	***
Other	2.1% (0.5%)	2.7% (0.8%)	2.3% (0.7%)	1.5% (0.5%)			
Education							
Less than high school	46.1% (1.7%)	40.4% (2.4%)	47.2% (2.7%)	49.3% (1.9%)	*	**	
High school	30.6% (1.3%)	32.8% (2.8%)	29.9% (2.1%)	29.5% (1.3%)			
More than high school	23.4% (1.2%)	26.9% (2.2%)	22.9% (2.2%)	21.3% (1.3%)		*	
Marital Status							
Married (or partnered)	52.7% (1.4%)	64.7% (2.8%)	60.5% (2.7%)	40.9% (1.5%)		***	***
Divorced/ separated	11.2% (1.0%)	21.2% (2.3%)	10.8% (1.8%)	4.7% (0.8%)	**	***	**

(*continued on next page*)

TABLE 5.1. *(continued)*

Respondent Characteristics	All Ages (n = 2,559)	50–64 (LM) (n = 612)	65–74 (YO) (n = 540)	75+ (OO) (n = 1,107)	Significant Difference? LM vs. YO	LM vs. OO	YO vs. OO
Widowed	32.9% (1.0%)	10.2% (1.2%)	25.3% (2.2%)	51.8% (1.4%)	***	***	***
Never married	3.2% (0.5%)	3.8% (1.1%)	3.5% (1.0%)	2.6% (0.6%)			
Insurance[a]							
Medicare (1/0)	79.3% (1.1%)	39.1% (2.7%)	96.1% (1.0%)	97.8% (0.5%)	***	***	
Medicaid (1/0)	20.8% (1.5%)	23.3% (2.1%)	24.9% (2.4%)	17.0% (2.1%)		*	**
Private (1/0)	30.0% (1.4%)	42.5% (2.4%)	26.1% (2.5%)	23.7% (1.9%)	***	***	
No insurance (1/0)	3.1% (0.4%)	8.9% (1.2%)	1.3% (0.5%)	0.2% (0.0%)	***	***	
Currently Working	6.9% (0.7%)	15.7% (2.1%)	4.6% (1.0%)	2.2% (0.5%)	***	***	
Household Income[a]							
Quintile 1	41.2% (1.4%)	39.4% (3.0%)	41.0% (2.6%)	42.6% (1.6%)			
Quintile 2	25.8% (1.0%)	14.7% (1.7%)	29.9% (2.4%)	31.2% (1.6%)	***	***	
Quintile 3	14.9% (0.9%)	17.1% (1.8%)	13.5% (1.3%)	14.2% (1.2%)			
Quintile 4	10.3% (0.9%)	15.5% (1.8%)	9.3% (1.3%)	7.4% (0.9%)	***	***	
Quintile 5	7.8% (0.8%)	13.3% (2.1%)	6.4% (1.3%)	4.7% (0.6%)	**	***	

Note. LM = late middle age; YO = young old; OO = older old.
[a]Insurance categories are not mutually exclusive.
*$p < .05$. **$p < .01$. ***$p < .001$.

Similar proportions of all three age groups had never married, but though the late-middle-aged and young old groups were equally likely to be married at the time of the survey (64.7% and 60.5%, respectively), they were both more likely to be married than the older old group (40.9%, $p < .001$). The proportion divorced decreased sharply and steadily with age from 21% among those in late middle age to 5% among those who were older old ($p < .001$), while widowhood increased by age in a similar manner from 10% among those in late middle age to 52% among the older old group ($p < .001$).

Individuals in late middle age and those who were young old were equally likely to receive Medicaid, accounting for almost a quarter of both groups. They were significantly more likely than the older old group to do so. The young old group did not differ from the older old group on any other health insurance indicator, however. Because of near-universal Medicare coverage at age 65, those in late middle age were less likely than their older counterparts to have Medicare, although 39% of this group were medically eligible and did receive the benefit, and they were significantly more likely to be privately insured or uninsured altogether compared with the older old group.

Individuals in late middle age were more likely to be working (15.7%) than either those who were young old (4.6%, $p < .001$) or older old (2.2%, $p < .001$), who did not differ from one another. Finally, 40% of each age group fell into the lowest income quintile. But while individuals who received care had smaller incomes than the general population, those who were in late middle age were more than twice as likely as either the young old or older old group to fall within the highest quintile (13.3% vs. 6.4% and 4.7%, respectively, $p < .001$), likely partly reflecting their higher likelihood of currently working.

RESPONDENT CASEMIX

Table 5.2 examines respondent casemix among individuals who received at least some assistance. Here, individuals that were in the late-middle-aged, young old, and older old groups and received help with at least one ADL or IADL were more comparable in their health and functional statuses than were those in the previous chapter, which included respondents who reported having difficulty performing ADLs or IADLs regardless of whether or not they received any assistance. Like the previous sample, the average number of IADL difficulties increased significantly with age from 1.57 for individuals in late middle age, 1.74 for those who were young old, to 2.17 for those who were older old, while mean ADL difficulties were comparable for each group. There were no differences in the average number of days spent in the hospital over the previous 2 years, but the late-middle-aged and young old groups spent more days in bed over the past 30 days, on average, than did the older old group. Each group was equally likely to report the use of a wheelchair, but those in late middle age were more likely than either the young old or older old groups to report feeling extremely exhausted or fatigued over the past 2 weeks (55.4% vs. 44.6% and 42.9%, $p < .001$). Diagnosed psychiatric problems decreased significantly by age, accounting for 42% among late-middle-aged individuals, 29% among those who were young old, and 24% among those who were older old. Alternatively, cognitive impairment increased significantly by age from 7% among late-middle-aged adults, 17% among those who were young old, and 25% among those who were older old.

The proportion of individuals from the sample who were morbidly obese, defined as having a BMI of greater than 40, dropped significantly by age, accounting for 13% of those in late middle age, 7% of the young old group, and <1% of the older old group.

Table 5.2. Respondent casemix by age group for individuals who receive help with at least one ADL or IADL.

Respondent Characteristics	All Ages (*n* = 2259)	50–64 (LM) (*n* = 612)	65–74 (YO) (*n* = 540)	75+ (OO) (*n* = 1,107)	Significant Difference? LM vs. YO	LM vs. OO	YO vs. OO
Number of ADL Difficulties (*M, SE*)	1.86, .05	1.93, .08	1.86, .08	1.81, .07			
Number of IADL Difficulties (*M, SE*)	1.89, .05	1.57, .05	1.74, .08	2.17, .06	*	***	***
Number of Hospitalizations in Past 2 Years (*M, SE*)	6.81, .42	5.98, .63	7.89, .73	6.83, .75			
Number of Bed Days in Past Month (*M, SE*)	3.77, .23	4.67, .43	4.27, .49	2.90, .28		***	**
	% (*SE*)	% (*SE*)	% (*SE*)	% (*SE*)			
Easily Fatigued/Exhausted in Past 2 Weeks	47.1% (1.1%)	55.4% (1.9%)	44.6% (1.9%)	42.9% (1.6%)	***	***	
General Health							
Excellent	2.2% (0.4%)	2.5% (0.9%)	1.6% (0.5%)	2.4% (0.4%)			
Very good	7.3% (0.6%)	4.8% (1.2%)	5.3% (1.1%)	10.0% (1.0%)		**	**
Good	21.1% (1.0%)	16.5% (1.9%)	21.1% (2.1%)	24.3% (1.4%)		**	
Fair	32.3% (1.1%)	32.3% (2.6%)	31.3% (2.5%)	32.7% (1.7%)			
Poor	37.1% (1.2%)	44.0% (2.1%)	40.8% (2.5%)	30.5% (1.%)		***	***
Wheelchair Use	11.9% (0.8%)	10.4% (1.8%)	12.7% (1.6%)	12.6% (1.1%)			
Psychological Disorder	30.6% (1.3%)	42.4% (2.6%)	28.6% (2.2%)	23.7% (1.3%)	***	***	*

(*continued on next page*)

TABLE 5.2. *(continued)*

Respondent Characteristics	All Ages (n = 2259)	50–64 (LM) (n = 612)	65–74 (YO) (n = 540)	75+ (OO) (n = 1,107)	Significant Difference? LM vs. YO	LM vs. OO	YO vs. OO
Cognitive Impairment	17.6% (0.9%)	7.0% (1.1%)	16.9% (2.1%)	25.0% (1.6%)	***	***	**
Pain	59.5% (1.1%)	72.7% (2.1%)	59.2% (2.2%)	50.7% (1.4%)	***	***	***
Number of Medical Conditions (*M, SE*)	2.92, 0.03	2.85, 0.08	3.02, 0.07	2.90, 0.06			
Body Mass Index							
Underweight (BMI < 18.5)	5.2% (0.5%)	2.2% (0.9%)	5.4% (1.2%)	7.1% (0.9%)	*	***	
Normal/obese	88.8% (0.7%)	84.7% (1.9%)	87.6% (1.6%)	92.2% (0.9%)		**	*
Morbidly obese (BMI > 40)	6.0% (0.6%)	13.1% (1.5%)	7.0% (1.3%)	0.7% (0.3%)	**	***	***

Note. LM = late middle age; YO = young old; OO = older old.
*p < .05. **p < .01. ***p < .001.

At the other end of the weight spectrum, the proportion of those who were considered underweight, with a BMI less than 18, was similar among the young old and older old groups (5.4% and 7.1%), both of which were significantly higher than the late-middle-aged group (2.2%). Finally, in general, both late-middle-aged and young old adults were more likely to consider themselves in poor health compared with their older old counterparts.

Care Networks

Table 5.3 presents care network characteristics by age group. The structure of the care networks of the late-middle-aged and young old groups was strikingly similar, although a few differences did emerge. Young old adults were less likely than those who were in late middle age to have had an unpaid nonrelative in their care network (4.3% vs. 10.2%, $p < .01$) though they were three times as likely as the late-middle-aged group to have supplemented informal help with formal help (9.9% vs. 3.2%, $p < .01$). They were also more likely than the late-middle-aged group to have named a formal caregiver as their primary caregiver (8.9% vs. 5.6%, $p < .05$), but they were equally likely to have had formal care as their sole source of care (4.8% and 4.2%).

Because of the similarities between individuals who were in the late-middle-aged and young old groups, the remaining comparisons are made between the late-middle-aged and older old groups only, but hold for the young old group as well unless otherwise noted. Close to 70% of individuals in late middle age relied on the support of only one helper (67.8%). This was significantly higher than the percentage of those who were older old who did so (53.2%, $p < .001$). Forty-five percent of individuals in late middle age were cared for solely by a spouse, much higher than the only 27% of the older old group ($p < .001$).

TABLE 5.3. Care network characteristics by age group of individuals who receive help with at least one ADL or IADL.

Respondent Characteristics	All Ages (n = 2,259)	50–64 (LM) (n = 612)	65–74 (YO) (n = 540)	75+ (OO) (n = 1,107)	Significant Difference? LM vs. YO	LM vs. OO	YO vs. OO
Number of Caregivers (*M, SE*)	1.70, .02	1.55, .04	1.63, .04	1.84, .04		***	***
	% (*SE*)	% (*SE*)	% (*SE*)	% (*SE*)			
Has Only 1 Caregiver	59.9% (1.2%)	67.8% (1.9%)	62.9% (2.5%)	53.2% (1.8%)		***	***
Mixture of Care (1)							
Spouse only	35.6% (1.1%)	45.0% (2.1%)	40.8% (2.9%)	26.8% (1.5%)		***	***
Informal only (may include spouse)	47.9% (1.2%)	47.6% (2.0%)	44.6% (2.9%)	49.8% (1.8%)			
Formal only	5.4% (0.6%)	4.2% (0.9%)	4.8% (1.3%)	6.6% (0.8%)		*	
Bother formal and informal	11.0% (1.2%)	3.2% (0.8%)	9.9% (1.8%)	16.9% (2.0%)	**	***	**
Mixture of Care (2)							
Has a spouse caregiver (1/0)	46.5% (1.2%)	58.5% (2.7%)	53.4% (2.7%)	35.0% (1.4%)		***	***
Has a child caregiver (1/0)	43.7% (1.2%)	35.3% (2.1%)	39.4% (2.7%)	51.6% (1.6%)		***	***

Has either spouse or child caregiver (1/0)	82.7% (0.9%)	83.4% (2.3%)	84.7% (1.9%)	81.2% (1.0%)			
Has an "other" relative caregiver (1/0)	15.5% (1.1%)	13.7% (1.9%)	17.1% (1.9%)	15.9% (1.3%)			
Has a nonrelative caregiver (1/0)	7.6% (0.7%)	10.2% (1.9%)	4.3% (0.9%)	7.6% (0.7%)	**		**
Has a formal caregiver (1/0)	16.5% (1.1%)	7.4% (1.1%)	14.7% (1.7%)	23.4% (1.9%)	**	***	**
Relation of Primary Caregiver to Respondent							
Spouse	44.3% (1.2%)	56.5% (2.7%)	50.6% (2.9%)	32.9% (1.4%)		***	***
Child/(in-law)	31.5% (1.1%)	23.6% (1.9%)	29.4% (2.5%)	38.0% (1.5%)		***	**
Other relative	8.8% (0.7%)	8.5% (1.4%)	8.9% (1.5%)	8.9% (0.8%)			
Nonrelative	4.3% (0.6%)	5.8% (1.6%)	2.2% (0.7%)	4.4% (0.6%)			*
Formal	11.1% (0.7%)	5.6% (0.9%)	8.9% (1.3%)	15.8% (1.2%)	*	***	***

Note. LM = late middle age; YO = young old; OO = older old.
$^{*}p < .05$. $^{**}p < .01$. $^{***}p < .001$.

A full 58% of individuals in late middle age had a spouse as part of their care network, versus 35% of the older old group ($p < .001$)—however, in both age groups, the spouse (if present) served as the primary caregiver.

Children were present in the care networks of 35% of the individuals in late middle age and a full half (51.6%) of those who were older old ($p < .001$). Due to the presence of a spouse, those who were in late middle age were less likely to have had a child as a primary caregiver compared with those who were older old (23.6% vs. 38.0%, $p < .001$). Over 80% of all age groups had at least a spouse or a child in their care network, but while 81% of individuals who were in late middle age and 80% of those who were young old named one or the other as their primary caregiver, individuals who were older old were significantly less likely to have done so (70.9%, $p < .001$).

As table 5.3 also makes clear, the use of formal care increased with age. Twenty-three percent of individuals who were older old used at least some formal care compared with only 7% of the late-middle-aged and 15% of the young old groups. Nearly 7% of the older old group (6.6%) relied solely on formal care compared with only 4% of the late-middle-aged ($p < .01$) and 5% of the young old groups. It is striking, however, that while individuals in late middle age were much less likely to use formal assistance, over 50% of those who used it relied on it as their sole source of care, compared with only one-third of those who were young old and less than one-third of those who were older old who did so.

Age Differences in Network Composition in Light of Respondent Casemix

Do the age differences reported in table 5.3 hold when casemix is controlled? In other words, were there cohort and life stage

TABLE 5.4. Age differences in the likelihood of having particular care network characteristics.

	No. of Children β (*SE*)[a]	Spouse OR (*SE*)[b]	Nonrelative OR (*SE*)[b]	Formal Care OR (*SE*)[b]	Any Secondary Caregivers OR (*SE*)[b]
Age (ref: 75+)					
50–64	–0.14 (0.04)**	2.44 (0.31)***	1.35 (0.34)	0.26 (0.06)***	0.65 (0.10)**
65–74	–0.12 (0.04)**	2.05 (0.28)***	0.54 (0.14)*	0.59 (0.11)**	0.78 (0.10)
N	2,161	2,161	2,161	2,161	2,161
***F*(*nDF*, *dDF*)**	(15, 38) = 8.91	(15, 38) = 8.12	(15, 38) = 2.67	(15, 38) = 22.74	(15, 38) = 22.02
prob. > *F*	0.0000	0.0000	0.0074	0.0000	0.0000

Note. Models control for respondent casemix. OR = odds ratio.
[a]OLS regression.
[b]Logistic regression.
$^*p < .05$. $^{**}p < .01$. $^{***}p < .001$.

differences in the composition of the care networks independent of the need for care? Table 5.4 presents age differences in the likelihood of having various network characteristics after controlling for casemix.

As is evident, age differences in care network composition persisted. Individuals in both the late-middle-aged and young old groups were more likely to have had a spouse in their care networks and less likely to have had children compared with their older old counterparts. Those who were young old had fewer nonrelatives in their networks compared with either individuals who were older old or in late middle age who did not differ from one another. Individuals in both the late-middle-aged and young old groups were less likely than those who were older old to have had any formal caregivers in their networks, although those who were young old were significantly more likely than those who were in late middle age to have done so. Finally, the late-middle-aged and the young old groups were less likely than the older old group to have reported any secondary caregivers.

DISCUSSION

Even after controlling for casemix, the care networks of individuals who were in the late-middle-aged and young old groups were very different from the networks of the older old. They were smaller in size, dominated by spousal care, and primarily informal. Less than 10% of those in late middle age used formal care at all. For all groups, however, spouses and children constituted the majority of primary caregivers.

All else being equal, given the composition of the care networks presented in this chapter, one might be tempted to suggest that younger groups were actually better off than the older old group in terms of getting the care that they needed. After all, like those who were older old, at least 80% of individuals in both the young old and late-middle-aged groups had children and/or spouses in their care networks, and they were significantly more likely than those who were older old to have named one or the other as their primary caregiver. Spouses, in particular, the group that has historically been shown to provide the most overall care, were more prevalent in the care networks of the late-middle-aged and young old groups compared with the older old group. This is precisely why researchers must consider the life stage and cohort differences of both the care receivers and care givers. The remaining chapters explore this next step. Given casemix, demographic characteristics of the respondent, and care network characteristics, the remaining chapters examine whether the number of hours that individuals in late middle age received in assistance per month differed from that received by those who were older old. They demonstrate that differences in hours of care by age were associated not only with the characteristics of the respondent and care network as a whole but with those of the caregiver as well.

Chapter 6

Hours of Care

For the remaining analyses, we examined age differences in the amount of care respondents received, given at least a minimal amount of care. Though no one really knows how much care is truly enough or too much, LaPlante et al. (2004) demonstrated that a shortfall in hours was associated with negative health and utilization outcomes. In a study of adults with functional limitations, they found that individuals with two or more unmet ADL needs were more likely than those without to experience negative consequences, including discomfort, weight loss, dehydration, falls, burns, and dissatisfaction with the help received. Therefore, it was critical for us to examine not only who received care and from whom but also the amount of care received.

The life course perspective suggests that many different factors influence the amount of care an individual receives.

These factors include not only the characteristics of the individual receiving help but also the characteristics of his or her care network, as well as the characteristics of the individuals who make up the care network. We demonstrate that even when the structure of the care network is similar (e.g., network size and/or relation of primary caregiver to respondent), differences across age groups remain. In this and the following chapter, we explore the remaining age difference in hours of care by examining the characteristics and competing responsibilities of individual caregivers, specifically the two most common caregivers (spouses and children). We demonstrate that much of the remaining age differences in hours of care were explained by the characteristics of the individuals who provided that care.

Bivariate Relationship Between Hours of Care and Age

Figure 6.1 displays the bivariate relationship between hours of care and age for total care, care provided by the primary caregiver, and care provided by secondary helpers. These bivariate relationships indicate that there were clear age differences in the receipt of care, with late-middle-aged individuals receiving the fewest hours of care overall, despite the discovery that over half of them had their spouse as their primary caregiver (as seen in the previous chapter). We also see that the shortfall in hours given by the primary caregiver to those who were in late middle age was not compensated for by the care provided by supplemental caregivers. Rather, there also appears to have been a shortfall in secondary hours of care between those in late middle age and their older counterparts.

FIGURE 6.1. Bivariate relationship between age and hours of care.

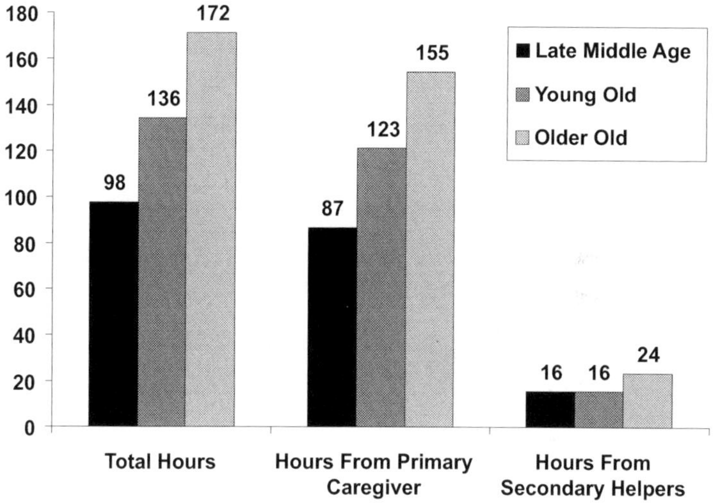

MULTIVARIATE RESULTS

OLS regression analyses were carried out on both logged total hours of care provided by the care network and logged hours provided by the primary caregiver, but since the results are almost identical, this discussion focused on hours of care provided by the primary caregiver. We chose primary caregiver hours over total hours because (a) a majority of individuals have only one caregiver, and (b) the discussion frames the next chapter, which looks individually at the two most prominent primary caregivers: spouses and children. Appendix C provides the OLS regression models for total hours of care not reported here.

Main effects results are displayed in table 6.1, followed by results of significant age interactions in table 6.2. We formally

TABLE 6.1. OLS regression of logged hours of care from a primary caregiver in the past month.

	β (*SE*)
Constant	3.33 (0.19)***
Age (ref: 75+)	
50–64	–0.38 (0.10)***
65–74	–0.23 (0.10)*
Currently Working	–0.30 (0.14)*
Male	–0.25 (0.07)***
Lives Alone	–0.76 (0.10)***
Education (ref: high school)	
Less than high school	–0.06 (0.08)
More than high school	0.02 (0.09)
Race/Ethnicity (ref: non-Hispanic White)	
Non-Hispanic Black	–0.04 (0.10)
Hispanic	0.25 (0.16)
Other	0.05 (0.23)
Household Income (ref: lowest quintile)	
Quintile 2	0.15 (0.12)
Quintile 3	0.07 (0.11)
Quintile 4	–0.03 (0.13)
Quintile 5	–0.17 (0.14)
Number of Informal Caregivers	0.15 (0.03)***
Primary Caregiver (ref: spouse)	
Child	–0.30 (0.09)***
Other relative	–0.44 (0.13)***
Nonrelative	–0.54 (0.20)**
Formal	–0.13 (0.17)
Receives Any Formal Assistance	0.33 (0.12)**
N, R^2	2,156, .34
$F(nDF, dDF)$	(33, 20) = 38.51
prob. > F	0.0000

Note. All models control for respondent casemix (number of ADL difficulties, number of IADL difficulties, number of nights in hospital, fatigue, number of days in bed, wheelchair use, general health, presence of a psychological disorder, pain, number of medical conditions, and body mass index).
$*p < .05$. $**p < .01$. $***p < .001$.

TABLE 6.2. OLS regression of logged hours of care received in the past month from a primary caregiver with age interactions.

	Model 1 β (*SE*)	Model 2 β (*SE*)
Constant	3.24 (0.17)***	3.34 (0.19)***
Age (ref: 75+)		
50–64	−0.27 (0.12)*	−0.43 (0.10)***
65–74	0 (0.13)	−0.21 (0.10)*
Primary Caregiver (ref: spouse)		
Child	−0.12 (0.11)	−0.31 (0.09)***
Other relative	−0.12 (0.20)	−0.44 (0.13)***
Nonrelative	−0.56 (0.21)*	−0.54 (0.20)**
Formal	0.02 (0.21)	−0.17 (0.17)
Receives Any Formal Assistance	0.30 (0.12)*	0.31 (0.12)*
Age × Primary Caregiver Interaction (ref: older old, spouse)		
50–64 × Child	−0.31 (0.16)	
50–64 × Other relative	−0.53 (0.26)*	
50–64 × Nonrelative	0.28 (0.47)	
50–64 × Formal	0.29 (0.29)	
65–74 × Child	−0.34 (0.17)	
65–74 × Other relative	−0.58 (0.37)	
65–74 × Nonrelative	−0.43 (0.63)	
65–74 × Formal	−0.58 (0.25)*	
Age × Formal Care Interaction (ref: older old, no formal care)		
50–64 × Formal care		0.53 (0.22)*
65–74 × Formal care		−0.16 (0.20)
***N*, R^2**	2,156, .34	2,156, .34
***F*(*nDF*, *dDF*)**	(41,12)	(35, 18)
prob. > F	0.0000	0.0000

Note. Model controls for all variables included in table 6.1.
**p* < .05. ***p* < .01. ****p* < .001.

tested age interactions with three care network variables—relation of primary caregiver to the respondent, whether or not the respondent received any formal care, and number informal helpers. Each variable was tested separately so as not to overload the model, and only significant interactions were reported.

We interpreted coefficients derived from a log-transformed dependent variable as $100(\beta)$ = percent change in *Y* given a unit increase in *X*. With this in mind, we see in table 6.1 that after controlling for both casemix and sociodemographic characteristics, the structure of the social network was significantly associated with hours of care. Having a greater number of informal caregivers in the network was associated with more hours of help provided by the primary caregiver. More specifically, the presence of each additional informal caregiver was associated with a 15% increase in the hours provided by the primary caregiver. This positive relationship between the number of caregivers and the hours of care suggests that individuals relied on secondary caregivers not to ease the general burden of the primary caregiver, but rather to fulfill a need that went beyond the capabilities of one person.

The relationship of the primary caregiver to the respondent was also significantly associated with hours of care, although the nature of this relationship differed somewhat by age, as model 1 in table 6.2 suggests. As expected, the main effects model indicates that child, "other relative," and nonrelative primary caregivers provided fewer hours of care than did spousal caregivers—and this relationship is maintained across all age groups. Other relative primary caregivers to individuals in late middle age, however, provided even fewer hours of care compared with spousal caregivers than did other relative caregivers to those who were older old ($p < .05$; see model 1 in table 6.2). The interaction of age and formal primary caregiver showed that while, generally speaking, there was no difference in the hours of care provided by formal primary caregivers compared with spousal primary caregivers between the late-middle-aged and older old groups, formal primary caregivers to those who were young old provided fewer hours of care compared with spousal caregivers than did formal caregivers of the older old group ($p < .05$).

Age differences in the relationship between any formal care (whether the formal caregiver was primary or secondary) and logged hours of care by the primary caregiver were also significant (see model 2 of table 6.2). In general, the receipt of any formal care was associated with greater hours of care provided by the primary caregiver. This positive relationship between formal care and hours received was even stronger for individuals in late middle age compared with those who were older old ($p < .05$). There was no significant difference, however, in the relationship between formal care and hours received between the young old and older old groups.

Discussion

The results of our analyses of hours of care provided by the primary caregiver clearly indicate that care network structure did matter, and also that the relationship between network structure and hours of care differed somewhat by age. The most striking interaction was the receipt of any formal assistance and age on hours of care. In this instance, the use of any formal care by individuals in late middle age, but not those who were young old, was associated with more hours of care provided by the primary caregiver when compared with those who were older old, suggesting that formal services were not substituting for family care in this population but were complementing the efforts of caregivers when care needs were high.

Individuals in late middle age were much less likely to receive care from formal caregivers than were individuals who were older old, but when they did receive such care, they were more likely to rely solely on it as we found in the previous chapter. When formal care was used by late-middle-aged adults, it was likely used as a method of last resort to fulfill a need that informal care could not. That those who were young old did not differ from older old adults in this regard is noteworthy and lends support to the notion that formal services are more readily available to individuals over 65, although results do indicate that when formal care served as the primary caregiver to the young old group, it resulted in fewer hours of care for them compared with the older old group.

Despite the strong relationship between the structure of the care network and hours of care for late-middle-aged adults, the addition of these variables did not eliminate the age difference in hours of care between them and the older old group. However, we have not yet considered the importance of the characteristics of the caregivers themselves to hours of care. That is, given similar need and care structures, why did a spousal or child primary caregiver provide fewer hours to late-middle-aged adults than to older old adults? The next chapter examined whether the characteristics and competing demands of caregivers to those in late middle age limited the number of hours of care they had to give, thus explaining the remaining age difference in hours of care by the primary caregiver.

Chapter 7

Spouses and Children as Primary Caregivers

The relationship between two individuals is affected by the characteristics of both members, in this case the caregiver and the care recipient (Faber & Wasserman, 2001). In this chapter, we examine hours of care provided specifically by the two most important primary caregivers—spouses and children. In separate analyses, we considered the specific characteristics of each in order to try to explain the remaining age differences.

Differences in Respondent Characteristics by Primary Caregiver Type

It is first informative to know whether spouses provide care to a different type of respondent than children and other primary caregivers. Tables 7.1 and 7.2 present respondent sociodemographic,

TABLE 7.1. Respondent characteristics by primary caregiver (PC) type.

Respondents	Spouse PC (S) (*n* = 1,001)	Child PC (C) (*n* = 721)	Other PC (O) (*n* = 537)	Significant Difference?		
				S vs. C	S vs. O	C vs. O
Age (*M, SE*)	68.57 (0.43)	74.74 (0.55)	74.87 (0.78)	***	***	
	% (*SE*)	**% (*SE*)**	**% (*SE*)**			
Male	56.2% (1.7%)	17.1% (1.3%)	28.8% (2.2%)	***	***	***
Marital Status						
Married/partnered	—	16.2% (2.0%)	13.6% (1.9%)	—	—	
Divorced/separated	—	19.0% (1.8%)	21.6% (2.7%)	—	—	
Widowed	—	62.6% (2.3%)	54.5% (2.6%)	—	—	*
Never married	—	2.2% (0.8%)	10.3% (1.8%)	—	—	***
Race/Ethnicity						
Non-Hispanic White	82.1% (1.9%)	67.8% (2.4%)	65.6% (3.3%)	***	***	
Non-Hispanic Black	9.8% (1.5%)	18.0% (1.8%)	21.8% (2.7%)	***	***	*
Hispanic	6.5% (1.7%)	12.7% (2.5%)	9.3% (2.4%)	**	*	*
Other	1.6% (0.5%)	1.6% (0.6%)	3.4% (1.2%)			
Education						
Less than high school	36.3% (2.2%)	57.2% (2.2%)	49.4% (2.2%)	***	***	**

High school	34.3% (2.0%)	26.6% (1.8%)	28.9% (1.8%)	**	*	
More than high school	29.4% (1.5%)	16.2% (1.6%)	21.7% (2.2%)	***	**	*
Currently Works	10.8% (1.4%)	4.5% (0.8%)	3.0% (1.0%)	***	***	
Health Insurance						
Medicare	72.6% (1.7%)	84.0% (1.3%)	85.4% (2.4%)	***	***	
Medicaid	9.7% (1.4%)	26.9% (2.0%)	32.9% (2.7%)	***	***	*
Private	43.1% (2.0%)	18.0% (1.6%)	21.6% (2.4%)	***	***	
Uninsured	4.2% (0.8%)	2.8% (0.7%)	1.7% (0.8%)			
Household Income						
Quintile 1	14.7% (1.6%)	63.0% (2.0%)	61.5% (2.4%)	***	***	
Quintile 2	29.6% (1.5%)	24.2% (1.7%)	21.0% (2.2%)	*	**	
Quintile 3	23.3% (1.6%)	7.1% (1.1%)	9.8% (1.6%)	***	***	
Quintile 4	18.4% (1.5%)	3.6% (0.7%)	4.3% (1.0%)	***	***	
Quintile 5	14.1% (1.4%)	2.2% (0.7%)	3.4% (1.2%)	***	***	

*$p < .05$. **$p < .01$. ***$p < .001$.

casemix, and network characteristics by three primary caregiver types: spouses, children, and all others (i.e., other relatives, non-relatives, and formal help). Respondents cared for by spouses constituted the largest group, followed by those cared for by child primary caregivers. They were considerably younger and more likely to be male than respondents with child or other primary caregivers ($p < .001$). They were less racially diverse, better educated, more likely to be in the workforce, and had higher incomes than respondents cared for by child or other caregivers.

Respondents with child primary caregivers were more similar to those with other primary caregivers than they were to those with spousal primary caregivers, at least in terms of sociodemographic characteristics, although some differences were still apparent. They were less likely to be male or never married, and they were more likely to be widowed than respondents with other relative primary caregivers. Moreover, although respondents with child primary caregivers were more ethnically diverse than respondents with spousal caregivers, the racial/ethnic composition differed from respondents with other primary caregivers such that those with child primary caregivers were more likely to be Hispanic, while those with other primary caregivers were more likely to be Black. Finally, they were less well educated, but less likely to be on Medicaid than respondents with other relative primary caregivers.

Though the sociodemographic characteristics of respondents with spousal primary caregivers differed substantially from those with child primary caregivers, there was virtually no difference in respondent casemix between these two groups (see table 7.2). The only difference was that respondents with spousal caregivers have fewer IADL difficulties that those with child primary caregivers. Furthermore, both of these groups of respondents were

TABLE 7.2. Respondent casemix and network characteristics by primary caregiver (PC) type.

Respondents	Spouse PC (S) (*n* = 1,001)	Child PC (C) (*n* = 721)	Other PC (O) (*n* = 537)	Significant Difference?		
				S vs. C	S vs. O	C vs. O
Respondent Casemix						
Number of ADL Difficulties (*M, SE*)	1.79 (0.06)	1.72 (0.07)	2.17 (0.11)			***
Number of IADL Difficulties (*M, SE*)	1.66 (0.05)	1.98 (0.08)	2.17 (0.09)	***	***	*
Number of Nights in Hospital (*M, SE*)	6.15 (0.67)	7.28 (0.56)	7.43 (0.90)		***	
Number of Bed Days (*M, SE*)	3.88 (0.31)	3.49 (0.36)	3.92 (0.44)			
	% (*SE*)	**% (*SE*)**	**% (*SE*)**			
Fatigued	48.7% (1.6%)	49.7% (2.2%)	40.9% (2.9%)		*	*
Wheelchair	11.2% (1.2%)	11.0% (1.5%)	14.4% (1.5%)			
Psychological Disorder	29.7% (1.4%)	30.3% (1.9%)	32.7% (3.0%)			
Cognitive Impairment	15.2% (1.3%)	18.6% (1.8%)	20.5% (2.1%)			
Body Mass Index						
Underweight	4.2% (0.7%)	5.2% (1.0%)	7.1% (1.3%)			
Normal/obese	89.6% (1.2%)	90.2% (1.1%)	85.5% (1.7%)		*	*
Morbidly obese	6.2% (1.1%)	4.6% (0.9%)	7.4% (1.5%)			
Respondent's Care Network						
Secondary Caregivers	19.5% (1.7%)	43.5% (2.2%)	50.4% (2.5%)	***	***	
Any Formal Care	4.1% (0.9%)	7.8% (1.3%)	50.5% (2.6%)	**	***	***

$*p < .05$. $**p < .01$. $***p < .001$.

generally less impaired than respondents with other primary caregivers.

Finally, respondents with spousal primary caregivers were less likely than both respondents with child primary caregivers and those with other primary caregivers to have had any secondary caregivers or formal care.

CHARACTERISTICS OF SPOUSAL PRIMARY CAREGIVERS

As described in chapter 5, spousal primary caregivers comprised 56% of primary caregivers to individuals in late middle age, 51% to those who were young old, and 33% to those who were older old. By and large and regardless of age, when a spouse provided care, she or he served as the primary caregiver to the individual in need. Table 7.3 highlights age differences in select characteristics that may influence the amount of care that a spouse provides.

Though spousal primary caregivers did not differ in the average number of ADL or IADL difficulties that they themselves reported, spousal primary caregivers of late-middle-aged adults were less likely to also be receiving help with their own functional limitations compared with spousal primary caregivers of either young old ($p < .01$) or older old adults ($p < .05$). They were more likely to have other caregiving responsibilities than spouses of the older groups, with 38% caring for children under 18 and/or elderly parents compared with 12% of the spouses of the young old group ($p < .001$) and only 2% of spouses of the older old group ($p < .001$). Finally, over half (56.9%) of spousal primary caregivers of late-middle-aged adults were currently working, compared with 20% of the spousal caregivers to young old adults ($p < .001$) and 10% of the spousal primary caregivers to older old adults ($p < .001$).

TABLE 7.3. Characteristics of spousal primary caregivers by age group.

Spousal Primary Caregivers	All Ages (*n* = 1,001)	50–64 (LM) (*n* = 340)	65–74 (YO) (*n* = 297)	75+ (OO) (*n* = 354)	Significant Difference? LM vs. YO	LM vs. OO	YO vs. OO
	% (*SE*)	% (*SE*)	% (*SE*)	% (*SE*)			
Female	56.2% (1.7%)	51.6% (3.1%)	55.6% (3.4%)	62.0% (2.4%)		*	
Has Secondary Helpers	19.5% (1.7%)	20.3% (2.4%)	19.4% (2.5%)	18.8% (2.4%)			
Number of ADL Difficulties (*M*, *SE*)	0.34 (.02)	0.33 (0.05)	0.35 (0.06)	0.35 (0.05)			
Number of IADL Difficulties (*M*, *SE*)	0.20 (.02)	0.18 (0.02)	0.21 (0.04)	0.23 (0.04)			
	% (*SE*)	% (*SE*)	% (*SE*)	% (*SE*)			
Receives Help for Own Functional Limitations	10.5% (1.2%)	6.4% (1.6%)	13.2% (2.2%)	13.0% (2.2%)	*	*	
Cares for Either Parents or Dependent Children	18.6% (1.4%)	37.9% (2.2%)	11.5% (2.1%)	1.9% (0.7%)	***	***	***
Currently Works	30.9% (1.8%)	56.9% (2.9%)	19.6% (2.5%)	9.8% (1.7%)	***	***	**

Note. LM = late middle age; YO = young old; OO = older old.
*$p < .05$. **$p < .01$. ***$p < .001$.

SPOUSAL PRIMARY CAREGIVERS AND HOURS OF CARE

Figure 7.1 presents the bivariate relationship between hours of care provided by the spousal primary caregiver and age group. Spousal primary caregivers to late-middle-aged individuals, but not to those who were young old, provided fewer hours of care per month than spousal primary caregivers to those who were older old.

When respondent and household characteristics were controlled, the age difference that was demonstrated in the bivariate comparison remained, although it was substantially reduced (see model 1 in table 7.4). That is, spousal primary caregivers to late-middle-aged individuals provided fewer hours of care than those to older old individuals (marginally significant at $p = .06$),

FIGURE 7.1. Bivariate relationship between age and hours of care provided by spousal primary caregivers.

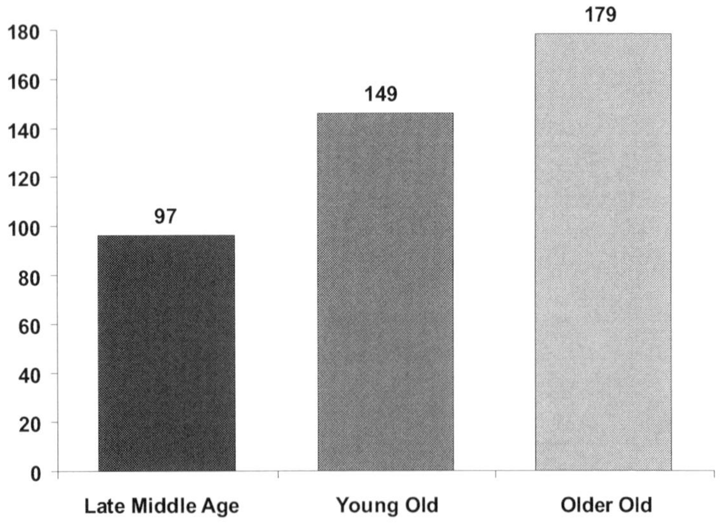

TABLE 7.4. Spousal primary caregiver—OLS regression of logged hours of care provided in past month.

	Model 1 β (*SE*)	Model 2 β (*SE*)	Model 3 β (*SE*)	Model 4 β (*SE*)
Constant	3.12 (0.32)***	3.38 (0.33)***	3.33 (0.33)***	3.30 (0.32)***
Age (ref: 75+)				
50–64	–0.24 (0.12)+	–0.29 (0.14)*	–0.13 (0.13)	–0.08 (0.12)
65–74	0.01 (0.13)	0 (0.13)	0.04 (0.13)	0.05 (0.12)
Spouse Characteristics				
Receives help with own ADL/IADLs		0.02 (0.20)	0.01 (0.20)	0 (0.21)
Female		–0.27 (0.10)**	–0.23 (0.10)*	–0.22 (0.1)*
Has secondary caregivers		0.5 (0.14)***	0.51 (0.14)***	0.51 (0.14)***
Number of ADL difficulties		0.14 (0.05)**	0.13 (0.05)*	0.12 (0.05)*
Number of IADL difficulties		–0.3 (0.12)*	–0.32 (0.13)*	–0.31 (0.13)*
Currently works			–0.36 (0.12)**	
Cares for children/elderly parents			–0.09 (0.14)	–0.08 (0.14)
Work Status (ref: doesn't work)				
Less than 20 hours per week				–0.1 (0.15)
20–39 hours per week				–0.23 (0.2)
40 or more hours per week				–0.52 (0.16)**
***N*, R^2**	971, .31	956, .35	956, .36	956, .36
***F*(*nDF*, *dDF*)**	(25, 29) = 21.67	(30, 24) = 15.87	(32, 22) = 13.86	(34, 20) = 17.48
prob. > *F*	0.0000	0.0000	0.0000	0.0000

Note. Model controls for respondent casemix and sociodemographic characteristics.
$^{+}p = .06$. $^{*}p < .05$. $^{**}p < .01$. $^{***}p < .001$.

but spousal primary caregivers to young old adults did not. The difference between the late-middle-aged and young old groups was also significant (not shown).

Models 2 through 4 in table 7.4 examine changes in the age effect upon adding spousal characteristics. We entered spousal characteristics in phases. First, based on the frequency of distributions in table 7.3, we did not expect that controlling for caregiver gender, functional status, the presence of secondary helpers, and whether or not the spouse received help for his or her own functional limitations would reduce the age effect. Rather, we anticipated that this would increase it somewhat, particularly given that individuals who received help with their own functional limitations may have provided less care to their spouses than those who did not. Results in model 2 indicate that the addition of these variables did indeed increase the age difference in hours of care between those who were in the late-middle-aged and older old groups, however there was no significant effect of a spousal primary caregiver's own receipt of care on hours of care in general.

Next, we expected that those who were currently working or those caring for other dependents may have provided fewer hours of care to their spouses, and that the addition of these variables in the model would reduce the effect of age on hours of care. As model 3 indicates, the effect of age was reduced—however, current work status alone, and not additional caregiving responsibility for dependent children or elderly parents, drove these findings. Those who were currently working provided significantly fewer hours of care to their spouses than those who were not currently working, thus explaining the remaining effect of age on hours of care.

Recall that 22% of spousal primary caregivers to young old adults worked, and yet there was no difference in hours of care provided compared with the spousal primary caregivers of the older old group even before work status was controlled. Model 4 suggests more specifically that it was not just working, but working full time or more that significantly reduced hours of care provided. Among spousal primary caregivers to late-middle-aged adults, nearly 50% worked at least full time (47.2%), compared with only 9% of spousal primary caregivers to young old adults and only 3% of spousal primary caregivers to older old adults (see figure 7.2).

Some have speculated that a caregiver may work full time or more hours in order to earn enough money to pay for formal care for their relatives in need (Soldo & Hill, 1995). At least for spouses of late-middle-aged adults in our study, this does not appear to be the case, as less than 2% of respondents with

FIGURE 7.2. Work status of spousal primary caregivers by age group.

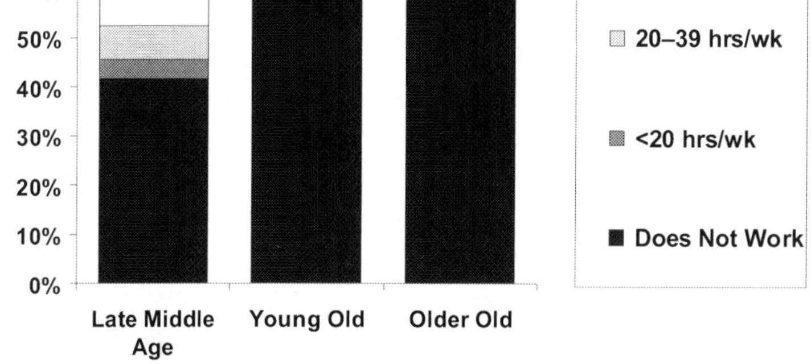

spousal primary caregivers who worked full time received any formal care at all in this study (results not shown).

More likely, spousal caregivers to adults in late middle age worked at least partly out of necessity. They were younger than the traditional retirement age, and if they had health insurance, it was likely to be employee-based health insurance (Weissman & Epstein, 1994). They were too young to qualify for Medicare, and even if their spouse requiring care met the strict health care cost and income criteria for Medicaid eligibility, insurance coverage did not extend to themselves or dependent children (Ho, Collins, Davis, & Doty, 2005).

CHARACTERISTICS OF CHILD PRIMARY CAREGIVERS

Children also play key caregiving roles for their parents. In this study, 25% of primary caregivers to late-middle-aged adults, 29% to young old adults, and 38% to older old adults were their children. Therefore, the sample size for these analyses was 721. The characteristics of these children are provided in table 7.5. The characteristics refer only to the child primary caregivers, not to all of the respondents' children.

As was expected, mean age of the child primary caregiver increased with respondent age group. Child primary caregivers of late-middle-aged adults were 31 years old on average, compared with 42 years among primary caregivers to young old adults and 54 years among the primary caregivers older old adults. There was no difference across age groups in the percentage who were male, which hovered around 30%. Almost 60% of child primary caregivers to those in late middle age had children of their own (58.1%), significantly less than the 70% of child primary caregivers to young old adults ($p < .05$) and 81% of child primary caregivers to older old adults ($p < .001$) who did so. There was

TABLE 7.5. Child primary caregiver characteristics by age group.

	All Ages (n = 712)	50–64 (LM) (n = 143)	65–74 (YO) (n = 146)	75+ (OO) (n = 423)	Significant Difference? LM vs. YO	LM vs. OO	YO vs. OO
Mean Age (*M, SE*)	46.12 (0.63)	30.54 (0.73)	42.78 (0.63)	54.27 (0.47)	***	***	***
	% (*SE*)	% (*SE*)	% (*SE*)	% (*SE*)			
Male	30.0% (2.1%)	29.7% (4.0%)	26.7% (4.3%)	31.5% (3.0%)			
Married	53.2% (2.6%)	34.6% (5.3%)	55.2% (4.3%)	60.2% (3.1%)	**	***	
Has Children	73.8% (1.9%)	58.1% (6.0%)	70.3% (4.8%)	80.8% (1.9%)	*	***	
Living Arrangement							
Lives with respondent	46.6% (2.3%)	49.7% (4.7%)	46.5% (4.9%)	45.4% (2.7%)			
Lives within 10 miles	30.1% (1.8%)	34.6% (4.9%)	26.8% (4.4%)	29.5% (1.8%)			
Lives > 10 miles	23.3% (1.8%)	15.7% (4.4%)	26.7% (4.2%)	25.1% (2.0%)			
Owns Home	47.4% (2.3%)	21.4% (4.0%)	46.5% (4.4%)	58.6% (2.5%)	**	***	*
Work Status							
Full time	53.2% (1.7%)	50.6% (4.3%)	61.9% (3.6%)	50.9% (2.3%)			*
Part time	3.7% (1.0%)	5.2% (1.8%)	11.4% (3.2%)	9.1% (1.3%)			
Does not work	35.2% (1.7%)	37.4% (4.0%)	26.8% (3.4%)	37.5% (2.1%)			**
Missing	3.0% (0.8%)	6.9% (2.9%)	0	2.6% (0.2%)	*		**

Note. LM = late middle age; YO = young old; OO = older old.
$^{*}p < .05$. $^{**}p < .01$. $^{***}p < .001$.

no significant difference across age groups in the percentage of child primary caregivers who lived with the respondent, lived within 10 miles of the respondent, or lived farther than 10 miles away.

The percentage of child primary caregivers who owned their own home increased significantly with age and was 21% among the child primary caregivers to individuals in late middle age, 47% among those to young old adults, and 59% among those to older old adults. Finally, primary caregivers to those who were young old were significantly more likely to be working full time and significantly less likely not to be working compared with primary caregivers to those who were older old. The work status of child primary caregivers to late-middle-aged adults was similar to that of child primary caregivers to older old adults.

CHILD PRIMARY CAREGIVERS AND HOURS OF CARE

Figure 7.3 presents the bivariate relationship between hours of care provided by the child primary caregiver and age group. Child primary caregivers to both late-middle-aged adults and young old adults provided fewer hours of care per month than child primary caregivers to older old adults. There was no significant difference between the hours provided by caregivers to the late-middle-aged and the young old groups.

As with the spousal analyses, respondent and household characteristics explained much of the age difference in hours of care provided to the young old and the older old groups, but the age difference in hours of care remained for the late-middle-aged group compared with the older old group (see model 1 in table 7.6). That is, controlling for respondent and household characteristics, child primary caregivers to individuals in late middle age provided significantly fewer hours of care than did those to older

FIGURE 7.3. Bivariate relationship between age and hours of care provided by child primary caregivers.

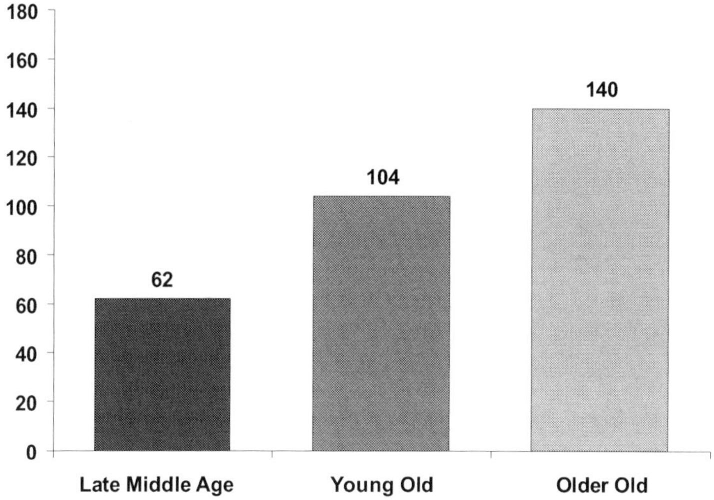

old adults, but child primary caregivers to young old adults did not. The difference in hours given by child primary caregivers to late-middle-aged and young old adults was not significant (not shown).

Unlike the spousal analyses, however, when child characteristics were added in model 2, a significant age difference between the young old and the older old groups in hours of care actually reappeared. One possible reason for this is that the child characteristics did not operate in the same way for each age. For instance, having children of their own may be more of an impediment to child primary caregivers of late-middle-aged adults versus older groups because these children are much younger and require more care themselves than do the presumably older children of the caregivers to the older age groups. Or, perhaps,

TABLE 7.6. OLS regression of logged hours of care from child primary caregivers.

	Model 1 β (*SE*)	Model 2 β (*SE*)
Constant	2.91 (0.35)***	2.59 (0.41)***
Age (ref: 75+)		
50–64	–0.42 (0.16)*	–0.53 (0.19)**
65–74	–0.26 (0.15)	–0.34 (0.13)*
Child Characteristics		
Has Secondary Helpers		0.30 (0.11)**
Work Status (ref: does not work)		
Full time		–0.14 (0.14)
Part time		–0.24 (0.16)
Missing		–0.03 (0.44)
Married		0.09 (0.12)
Male		–0.07 (0.11)
Owns own home		–0.13 (0.13)
Living Arrangement (ref: Lives > 10 miles)		
Lives with respondent		1.05 (0.13)***
Lives within 10 miles of respondent		0.45 (0.12)***
Has children		–0.09 (0.14)
***N*, *R*²**	673, .32	628, .40
***F*(*nDF*, *dDF*)**	(30, 27) = 20.51	(40, 14) = 8.81
prob. > *F*	0.0000	0.0000

Note. Models control for respondent casemix and sociodemographic characteristics.
*$p < .05$. **$p < .01$. ***$p < .001$.

full-time work status might operate differently for the younger caregivers compared with the older ones if there is a difference in the amount of flexibility their jobs allow. For instance, older adults are more likely to be in positions of authority at work and therefore more in control of their schedules, potentially allowing them to rearrange their time if their parent requires assistance. While the reasons themselves for potential age interactions cannot be tested in these analyses, we can at least determine whether child characteristics interacted significantly with respondent age group. We tested a series of models that included age interactions with each of the child characteristics. We tested the interactions separately in order not to overestimate the model resulting in seven interaction models, one for each child characteristic. Because the number of interactions increases the likelihood of finding a significant one, we used a Bonferroni adjustment that indicated that an interaction was significant only if it reached a significance level of $p < .007$ (.05/7). None of the interactions came close to that level of significance.

Discussion

Spousal Primary Caregivers

While spouses are often considered the optimal caregiver in time of need, these analyses suggest that the spouses of late-middle-aged adults may be less available than spouses of other age groups to provide assistance because of full-time work responsibilities. Research supports the finding that greater than part-time work results in fewer hours of care provided by a caregiver (Doty, Jackson, & Crown, 1998). Close to half of spousal primary caregivers of late-middle-aged adults worked 40 hours or more per week. This is in stark contrast to the 9% of spousal primary caregivers of young old adults and 3% of spousal primary caregivers of older old adults who did so.

Reasons for these work discrepancies by age of caregiver are easily identified. When an individual is caring for a functionally limited spouse, his or her income may be the sole income for the couple, making leaving or even limiting work impossible.

In addition, leaving one's employment to care for a spouse full time may jeopardize insurance coverage, a full pension due to retiring too early, and/or future social security benefits. These factors are particularly relevant to individuals under 65.

Child Primary Caregivers

Unlike the spousal analyses, the child characteristics tested here did not account for the age differences in the hours of care provided by child primary caregivers to their parents. In fact, they appeared to actually increase the differences. Additionally, child characteristics did not appear to affect hours of care differently by age group.

Clearly, the difference in hours of care by child primary caregivers to these three distinct age groups deserves further attention. First, it is possible that the measures themselves were not completely accurate. Spousal characteristics were obtained directly from the spouses themselves. Child characteristics, however, were obtained from the respondents and their proxies, when applicable. Measurement error is suggested in the measure of work status alone, where 7% of late-middle-aged adults could not state whether their child worked full time, part time, or not at all.

Another possibility is that the life stage variables considered here were not very important to the process compared with other variables. For instance, research indicates that children's motivations for caring are often complex. Affection toward a parent is associated with the provision of higher levels of care, as is the receipt of financial transfers from a parent earlier in life (Silverstein, Conroy, Wang, Giarrusso, & Bengston, 2002). Providing care for altruistic reasons (i.e., providing care to a parent in need simply because the parent needs help, rather than because it will benefit the caregiver in some way) increases with age (Silverstein et al., 2002), placing late-middle-aged adults at a disadvantage compared with older old adults in this regard. Affection toward parents and financial transfers from them early in life may also vary considerably across child caregiver cohorts. In these analyses, the child caregivers to older old adults included baby boomers and pre-boomers, the child caregivers of young old adults fell squarely within the baby boom generation, and the child caregivers of late-middle-aged adults were of the Generation X cohort. It is reasonable to expect that their childhood experiences differed, which may have influenced the relationships they had with their parents and ultimately the amount of care they were willing to provide them.

Still another possibility is that the desires of the care recipients themselves influenced the amount of care that their child provided. Perhaps, even at equal levels of need, individuals in late middle age who required assistance did not request or accept as much help from their children as they might have benefited from because they did not want to be considered a burden. Being functionally limited at their stage in life is not commonly considered part of the normal aging process, and they may have been less inclined than older old adults to accept help, or at least large amounts of help, from their children. Individuals who were older old, on the other hand, may have viewed their child's help as part of the normal circle of life.

All of these possibilities need to be explored with further research. Without a safety net of services available to those in late middle age, the need for assistance at this young age is likely to impose a great burden on both the care recipient and his or her children.

Chapter 8

Summary and Conclusion

Using the 2000 wave of the Health and Retirement Study, to our knowledge, we were the first to highlight the characteristics and community-based needs of people in late middle age with functional limitations. We exposed serious vulnerabilities in their potential support systems, and by doing so we demonstrated the importance of considering the life course, particularly the family resources and age-related public policies associated with younger and older stages of the life course, when studying community-based care.

In the area of informal caregiving, much attention has been given to (a) the concern for the growing numbers of individuals in late life who will need assistance as the large baby boom cohort ages, and (b) the plight of family caregivers (primarily women) who increasingly balance the demands of employment and informal caregiving to elderly parents. While both of these are important, exclusive focus on elderly persons and adult daughter caregivers has overshadowed the large group of individuals who are in need of care in late midlife. Our primary concern was to provide evidence of the disadvantage of being functionally limited in late middle life compared with later life, in terms of caregiving resources.

Summary of Findings

In chapter 4, we first described age differences in the characteristics of individuals who reported difficulty performing at least one ADL or IADL and found that individuals with functional limitations in late midlife looked very different from their older counterparts. We saw the demographic shifts in education, marital status, and race/ethnicity that occurred in the U.S. population as a whole over the latter half of the 21st century. Specifically, people in late middle age with functional difficulties were more highly educated than their older counterparts; younger groups were increasingly more likely to be single due to divorce or never having married, and both young old and late-middle-aged adults were more ethnically diverse than the older old. Finally, given the longer life expectancy of women, there were more men with difficulty in daily life activities within the younger versus older cohorts.

In terms of respondent casemix, although all groups showed similar levels of ADL impairment, late middle-aged adults were more likely than their older counterparts to be restricted to bed in the month prior to the survey, to have psychological disorders, to suffer from pain and fatigue, and to be morbidly obese. People in the older old cohort were more likely to report cognitive impairments and a higher level of hospitalizations, and a greater percentage were underweight compared to their younger counterparts. Adults who were young old shared a mix of characteristics with both age groups. The bottom line is that late-middle-aged, young old, and older old adults with difficulties in our study were very different groups of people, reflecting cohort differences, as well as differences in the nature of the health problem causing need for assistance. For example, people requiring care prematurely are more likely to suffer from injuries and musculoskeletal problems than people who are disabled "on time."

In chapter 4, we also saw that late-middle-aged adults were seemingly advantaged when considering their support networks. Though rates of divorce and never having married were high among late-middle-aged adults, nearly two-thirds were currently married, and they had larger family networks overall compared to their older counterparts. They were also just as likely as other groups to have an adult daughter in their support networks. And yet, both late-middle-aged and young old adults were less likely than those who were older old to receive any care from informal caregivers.

The difference was even more striking for formal care, where those who were young old were two times more likely and those who were older old four times more likely to receive any type of paid assistance compared to late-middle-aged adults. Though we did not have the statistical power to examine differences in formal care using multivariate methods, it is not difficult to see the current structure of our long-term care system reflected in the bivariate relationships. Formal care is largely unavailable to those in late middle age. It is prohibitively expensive to be paid for out-of-pocket, and eligibility for government-sponsored assistance is dependent upon age. It is also quite reasonable to deduce from the figures that late-middle-aged adults may be ill-informed about their formal care options. We saw that those with sisters (who may themselves have been caring for an elderly parent and therefore knowledgeable about long-term care services) appeared more likely to receive formal care than those without sisters. While obviously not conclusive in this study, the results deserve further attention.

In chapter 5, we examined the actual care networks of those who received at least a minimum amount of care. After controlling for respondent casemix, we found that the care networks of late-middle-aged and young old adults were smaller in size, dominated by spousal care, and primarily informal. Strikingly, while nearly one in four older old adults used at least some formal care, fewer than 1 in 10 late-middle-aged adults did so. For all groups, however, spouses and adult children still constituted the majority of primary caregivers.

Chapter 6 confirmed that even after controlling for the differing sociodemographic and casemix characteristics of the three groups, late-middle-aged and young old adults received fewer hours of care from their primary caregivers compared to those who were older old and that this reduction in hours of care was not supplemented by care from secondary caregivers. Keep in mind that we had already established that the younger groups were less likely than the older group to have a caregiver in the first place. Now, after limiting our sample to only those with at least one caregiver, we saw that late-middle-aged and young old adults were disadvantaged compared to those who were older old in the amount of care they received from their caregivers. Reasons for these discrepancies were examined in chapter 7. We examined spousal primary caregivers and adult child primary caregivers separately, as they constituted the majority of primary caregivers to all age groups.

Despite receiving fewer hours of care from their primary caregivers overall, those who were young old received as much care from their spousal primary caregivers as did older old adults. So, the shortcoming in hours of care that we observed in chapter 6 must be due to shortcoming in hours of care provided by other types of primary caregivers. Late-middle-aged adults, however, did not show the same pattern. Rather, they received fewer hours of care from their spousal primary caregivers than did both older groups. We demonstrated that this was primarily associated with the competing demands on the caregiver's time of full-time employment. Among spousal primary caregivers to late-middle-aged adults, nearly 50% were working at least full time while assuming primary caregiving responsibilities for their spouse. This was in contrast to 9% of spousal primary caregivers to those who were young old and only 3% of the spousal primary caregivers to those who were older old who were doing so. Unlike work responsibilities, neither the competing demands of dependent children nor caregiving to elderly parents had any effect on the hours of care given to a spouse.

After spouses, the next most reliable and important sources of care are the children of those in need. The analyses of child primary caregivers were not as straightforward. While it was clear that child primary caregivers to both late-middle-aged and young old adults provided fewer hours of care to their parents than did those to those who were older old, reasons for these differences were not uncovered here. The complexity of differences between the relationships of younger and older parent-child dyads were not captured by the measures used.

Life Course Perspective Revisited

Our study was heavily influenced by the life course perspective as described by Elder (1994) and others. Within the paradigm, emphasis is given to the importance of considering human lives within the context of their own developmental timing, the historical times in which they live, relationships they have with others, and their own human agency. Our results demonstrate nicely both the importance and the difficulty of considering these concepts when conducting social science research. Until now, the majority of our understanding about the care networks and experiences of adults with difficulties in function came from studies of the older population aged 65 and older. Similarly, our knowledge of caregiving stemmed from studies of care provided by elderly spouses or adult children to elderly parents. Without consideration of the life course, it is easy to generalize these findings to the care experiences of younger adult groups. However, these analyses demonstrate that people in late middle age with difficulties in function differ greatly from their older counterparts, as do the care networks of these groups. Furthermore, the older population themselves (aged 65 and older) are not a homogenous group. In our analyses, young old adults (65–74) and their care experiences differed substantially from older old adults (75 and older).

Life Course and People in Late Middle Age

Employment and marriage are two typical life situations of individuals in late midlife. A full 64% of individuals in late midlife with difficulties in function were married in our nationally representative sample. While spouses accounted for more than half of the primary caregivers of this age group, nearly half of those primary caregivers were working full time while serving as primary caregiver. Differences in the full-time work status of spousal primary caregivers explained much of the difference in informal hours of care received by late-middle-aged adults versus adults in the older age groups, as those who worked at least full time were likely to provide fewer hours of care than those who were not employed. This finding is supported by the literature, which states that although employment does not lessen the likelihood of becoming a caregiver (Moen, Robison, & Fields, 1994), women who are employed provide fewer hours of care to family in need than women who are not employed (Doty et al., 1998). The present findings generalize to both men and women and are particularly salient for those in late middle age, since they were more likely than their older counterparts to be cared for by a spouse.

Some have speculated that caregivers may work full-time or greater hours in order to earn enough money to pay for formal care for their relatives in need (Soldo & Hill, 1995). At least for this age group, this does not appear to be the case. Less than 2% of respondents with spousal primary caregivers who worked full time received any formal care at all (results not shown). More likely, spousal caregivers to late-middle-aged adults work at least partly out of necessity. This is particularly true of this cohort in the year 2000 in the United States. They are likely younger than the traditional retirement age, and if they have health insurance, it is likely to be employee-based health insurance (Weissman & Epstein, 1994). They are too young to qualify for Medicare, and if their spouses meet the strict health care cost and income criteria for Medicaid, their spouses may be covered, but they certainly are not (Ho et al., 2005). Social security benefits are generally not available to this group, and the likelihood of those in late middle age having the security of Medicare and Social Security, even when they reach the appropriate ages, is no longer a given. It is likely critical for many spousal primary caregivers in late midlife to remain in the workforce full time to ensure both present and future financial security.

Additionally, this shortfall in hours due to full-time employment by the spousal primary caregiver was not compensated by hours from secondary helpers. Eighty percent of spousal primary caregivers to late-middle-aged adults in this study were the sole care providers to their spouses. Of the 20% who did share caregiving responsibilities with at least one other person, those who worked full time provided more hours of care to their spouses than those who did not work full time (results not shown). Therefore, the use of additional caregivers in this case was more likely the result of the respondent's level of need rather than the spousal primary caregiver's work status.

Life Course and Young Old Adults

The primary motivation for this study was to learn about late-middle-aged adults with difficulties in function, and how their caregiving situations compared to their counterparts in old age. Since this study was conceptualized within the life course paradigm, it became clear to us that representing people over age 65 as a single group was actually misrepresenting the heterogeneity of experience in a later life context. Young old adults, as we have called them throughout, were 65–74 years old at the time of the study. They were conceptually distinct from their younger and older counterparts for a number of reasons. They had successfully aged into benefits of both Medicare and Social Security but were still young enough to be fully engaged in the workforce if they so chose. More so than their predecessors, they had experienced divorce, but they had also experienced widowhood to a greater extent than their younger counterparts. They were the parents of the baby boom generation, a group that has been transforming the social landscape since their arrival in the 1940s–1960s. Whether they and their care experiences would more closely resemble those of late-middle-aged or older old adults was not clear at the outset, but what was clear was that this group actually represented a transition phase in which one life stage progressed to the next. Some were also early adopters of social trends more often associated with the baby boom generation, for example, higher rates of divorce.

We made some interesting discoveries about young old adults. Similar to those who were in late middle age, they were less likely than older old adults to receive any care given difficulties in function. Likewise, they received fewer hours of care from their caregivers compared to older old adults. Unlike those in late middle age, however, they did not receive fewer hours of care than older old adults when their spouse was their primary caregiver. One explanation is that many fewer spousal primary caregivers to young old adults worked full time compared to their younger counterparts. This buffer, however, is likely to be lessened in the coming decades. Rising ages for social security benefits, recent increases in retirement ages, reductions in pensions and retiree health insurance benefits in companies nationwide, and increased life expectancies may influence, and in some cases force, the young old of the future to remain in the labor force longer and more closely resemble the current group of late-middle-aged adults.

A somewhat unexpected finding was the interaction between marital status and age and its effect on the likelihood of receiving any care. We found that those who were young old, but not those in late middle age, who were divorced or separated were much less likely than other groups to receive any care. Given that divorced and separated persons are unlikely to rely on their ex-spouses for assistance, adult children are the next likely option for this group. As parents of the baby boom generation, the young old had access to more children than the other two groups. Why this did not translate into more help is unclear. Is the finding reflective of an ideology regarding boomers' relationship with their parents? Or does it have little to do with the specific characteristics of the young old group and their children in the year 2000 and more to do with the age group itself? The data available to us did not present a ready answer to these questions. Whether this is a generational hiccup that will disappear or a more challenging deficiency in the care networks of young old adults deserves further attention.

STRENGTHS OF THE STUDY

This study has a number of strengths; most important among them are the use of the HRS, the use of the life course framework, and the focus on a previously understudied age group—persons in late middle age. The HRS is an ongoing study that replenishes its sample every 6 years to ensure a sample representative of the population 50 and older. It is rich in information on intergenerational exchanges and has improved its questions regarding the receipt of community-based care substantially since 1998. No other survey includes the level of detail on both family members and caregiving that the HRS provides.

Use of a life course framework has allowed us to tease apart the reasons for the discrepancies in care that we observed. We have reiterated the importance of family to caregiving across all groups in this study and have seen evidence of the influence of age-based policies on the care provided to people old enough to suffer the impact of chronic disease, but not old enough to benefit from societal supports in place for the older population. The life stage disparities in care observed in this study are attributable to not only differential access to formal care but also access to the financial and health insurance benefits for their loved ones who are charged with their care.

Most importantly, this study focused on a group of individuals whose needs are not yet on the radar screen as the country tries to brace itself for the aging of the baby boom. Yet there are already many baby boomers who are now in late midlife and require assistance due to functional limitations. Until now, our understanding of family and formal community-based care for people with chronic disease and impairments is in reference to the older population. We hope this study will mark the beginning of an expansion of knowledge to include the latter part of midlife, when the impact of chronic disease is a reality for many. Otherwise, our perceptions of the needs of the care available for those who need it will remain incomplete, even distorted.

Limitations of the Study

While the strengths of the study outweigh the limitations, the limitations are important to mention. First, this was a cross-sectional study. As such, we were unable to determine whether the documented shortfall in hours for late-middle-aged adults compared with older old adults resulted in negative outcomes. However, our intent was to identify potential discrepancies in care, and by doing so, to fill a large gap in knowledge that we and other researchers can begin to fill in now that the groundwork has been laid.

As is generally the case with studies based on secondary analyses of already collected data, our study would have been strengthened by the addition of variables that could increase the explanatory power of our findings. In particular, a measure of the need for any/additional assistance, as well as a separate measure of the desire for any/additional assistance, would greatly improve the type and quality of caregiving studies that could be conducted using the HRS. The addition of these two items would add the greatest benefit with the least burden. Given the number of items involved, a nuanced level of difficulty for each ADL and/or IADL would likely not be practical. And while a direct measure of the length of time an individual has been receiving care would be ideal, the HRS now has four completed waves of quality data on care networks that will enable an approximate measure of this important covariate for researchers as they begin to expand the body of knowledge developed by this study.

POLICY IMPLICATIONS

It is clear that people in late middle age are disadvantaged compared with older adults in terms of both the receipt of any community-based care and the amount of care that they receive. They are also less likely than young old and older old adults to have any form of health insurance (Pol et al., 2000), suggesting that required medical care and prescription drugs must be paid for out-of-pocket, thus restricting access to needed care (Schoen, Simantov, Duchon, & Davis, 2000). For those with chronic conditions, poor access to care can potentially increase risk for illness exacerbations, with the potential to accelerate functional decline and further intensify their medical and supportive care needs (Brown, Bindman, & Lurie, 1998; McWilliams, Zaslavsky, Meara, & Ayanian, 2003).

Extending Medicare benefits to those in late middle age has been considered (Johnson, Moon, & Davidoff, 2002; Moon, 2005; Shea, Short, & Powell, 2001). Better still would be a move to universal health insurance, which, as of this writing, is again on the national agenda as health care costs continue to soar. We hope that the exorbitant cost of today's health insurance premiums will convince the American public of the necessity of wide-sweeping health care reform, despite the failure of previous attempts, defeated in the end by the nation's historical reluctance to support equitable health reform (Quadagno, 2005).

In addition, many states are restructuring their Medicaid long-term care systems to provide more options for community-based services and supports, thus averting nursing home placement for those whose needs can be met in a less restrictive setting (Shirk, 2007). However, a major incentive driving Medicaid restructuring is cost savings, with a focus on contraction rather than expansion of the population eligible for coverage (Miller, 2005). It is highly unlikely that the rigid requirements of eligibility for Medicaid long-term care benefits will become more inclusive any time in the near future, or that any universal health care plan, even if enacted, will extend to long-term care services.

The emergence of the welfare state in the 1960s assigned age 65 as a marker between middle and old age, with the assumption that this age best captures the transition between vitality and vulnerability, thus sanctioning dependence on government insurance at age 65 but not 64 (Settersten, 2002). Today, the arbitrariness of this marker of old age is becoming increasingly clear, as active life styles continue for decades after age 65 for some, while for others, vulnerability begins earlier, with the onset of chronic disease or sudden injury (O'Rand, 2005). While increases in the age at which full social security benefits can be drawn reflects recognition of the extended vitality of the former segment of our population, little attention is focused on the earlier need for health-related assistance of the latter.

The results of this study provide evidence that age-based health and social policies result in disparities in receipt of community-based care for people with chronic illness in late middle age. While we do not provide evidence of the consequences of these disparities, adverse health, economic, and quality-of-life effects on this vulnerable subgroup of our population are possible. We know that people disadvantaged in life course capital, that is, stocks of social and economic resources inherited, attributed, and/or accumulated over the life span (O'Rand, 2005) are overrepresented among people who age early, and it is this same population likely to be most harshly affected by policies based on chronological age rather than need.

It is not only the people requiring care who are affected. Approximately 16 million adults provided care to family members in 2005 (Ho et al., 2005). These caregivers are more likely to be in poor health, miss work, and lack health insurance compared with noncaregivers (Ho et al.). It has been estimated that caregiving responsibilities resulted in $218 billion in lost wages by caregivers in 1997 alone (Holtz-Eakin, 2005). For caregivers of late-middle-aged adults, this may set them on a course of cumulative disadvantage for the rest of their lives.

We conclude that the onset of disability, frailty, and poor health is variable and not defined by chronological age. Life stages are fluid rather than fixed, and equitable policies must be designed to be responsive to those with health and supportive care needs, regardless of age. As baby boomers continue to advance into late middle age, we hope that the sheer size of the population calls attention to this reality.

Appendix A

Calculating Adjusted Odds Ratios From Two-Way Interactions

This example is based on Age × Marital Status in chapter 4, table 4.5.

Goal: *To determine the relative difference in the relationship between age and the receipt of care across levels of marital status.*

Coefficients of relevance

OR_1A_{LM} OR_2A_{YO} $OR_3A_{LM}M_D$ $OR_4A_{LM}M_W$ $OR_5A_{LM}M_N$ $OR_6A_{YO}M_D$ $OR_7A_{YO}M_W$ $OR_8A_{YO}M_N$

where	and
$OR_1 = .82$	$A_{LM} = 1$ and $A_{YO} = 0$ if late middle age
$OR_2 = .72$	$A_{LM} = 0$ and $A_{YO} = 1$ if young old
$OR_3 = .71$	$A_{LM} = 0$ and $A_{YO} = 0$ if older old
$OR_4 = .44$	
$OR_5 = .81$	$M_D = 0$ $M_W = 0$ $M_N = 0$ if married
$OR_6 = .28$	$M_D = 1$ $M_W = 0$ $M_N = 0$ if divorced/separated
$OR_7 = .82$	$M_D = 0$ $M_W = 1$ $M_N = 0$ if widowed
$OR_8 = .91$	$M_D = 0$ $M_W = 0$ $M_N = 1$ if never married

So, for age differences by marital status, the adjusted odds ratios are calculated by the following:

Late Middle Compared With the Older Old

Married: OR_1A_{LM} $= 0.82$

Divorced/separated: $OR_1A_{LM} \times OR_3A_{LM}M_D$ $= 0.82 \times 0.71 = 0.58$

Widowed: $OR_1A_{LM} \times OR_4A_{LM}M_W = 0.82 \times 0.44 = 0.36$
Never married: $OR_1A_{LM} \times OR_5A_{LM}M_N = 0.82 \times 0.81 = 0.66$

YOUNG OLD COMPARED WITH THE OLDER OLD

Married: $OR_2A_{YO} = 0.76$
Divorced/
separated: $OR_2A_{YO} \times OR_6A_{YO}M_D = 0.76 \times 0.71 = 0.21$
Widowed: $OR_2A_{YO} \times OR_7A_{YO}M_W = 0.76 \times 0.44 = 0.62$
Never married: $OR_2A_{YO} \times OR_8A_{YO}M_N = 0.76 \times 0.81 = 0.69$

In this example, if we consider the comparison of the likelihood of the receipt of care between the young old and the older old, we see that the young old are approximately one-fifth *as* likely or 79% *less* likely (OR = 0.21) to receive informal care than the older old if they are divorced.

Appendix B

Percentages and Standard Errors for Figures 4.2a–c, 4.3a–c, and 4.4a–c

Table B1. (From figure 4.2a.) Bivariate relationship between the receipt of any formal help and select sociodemographic characteristics for individuals who report difficulty performing at least one ADL or IADL—late-middle-aged adults.

	% (*SE*) With Any Formal Help		**% (*SE*) With Any Formal Help**
Gender		**Currently Working**	
Male	4.11% (0.85%)		
Female	2.90% (0.73%)	No	4.8% (0.74%)
		Yes	0.66% (0.52%)
Marital Status			
Married/partnered	1.30% (0.39%)	**Insurance**	
Divorced/separated	5.80% (2.08%)	*Medicare (1/0)*	
Widowed	16.09% (3.63%)	No	3.06% (0.70%)
Never married	2.25% (1.64%)	Yes	4.80% (1.23%)
Race/Ethnicity		*Medicaid (1/0)*	
Non-Hispanic White	2.45% (0.55%)	No	2.30% (0.54%)
Non-Hispanic Black	5.82% (2.00%)	Yes	9.79% (2.66%)
Hispanic	7.83% (2.96%)		
Other	2.83% (2.86%)	*Private (1/0)*	
		No	5.58% (1.04%)
Education		Yes	1.67% (0.60%)
Less than high school	5.54% (1.17%)		
High school	1.97% (0.78%)		
More than high school	3.21% (1.07%)		

(continued on next page)

TABLE B1. *(continued)*

	% (*SE*) With Any Formal Help		% (*SE*) With Any Formal Help
Insurance		**Household Income**	
Uninsured (1/0)			
No	3.64% (0.65%)	Quintile 1	6.80% (1.34%)
Yes	3.11% (2.10%)	Quintile 2	4.00% (1.81%)
		Quintile 3	1.78% (1.21%)
		Quintile 4	0.86% (0.62%)
		Quintile 5	1.44% (1.01%)

TABLE B2. (From figure 4.2b.) Bivariate relationship between the receipt of any formal help and select social network characteristics for individuals who report difficulty performing at least one ADL or IADL—late-middle-aged adults.

	% (*SE*) With Any Formal Help
Number of	
Daughters	
0	4.05% (1.32%)
1	3.96% (1.18%)
2	2.29% (0.78%)
3	0.79% (0.58%)
4 or more	7.17% (3.92%)
Sons	
0	2.22% (0.88%)
1	4.53% (1.04%)
2	3.05% (1.30%)
3	3.01% (1.25%)
4 or more	8.06% (4.55%)
Sisters	
0	1.41% (0.54%)
1	5.04% (1.25%)
2	1.77% (0.89%)

(continued on next page)

TABLE B2. *(continued)*

	% (*SE*) With Any Formal Help
Sisters	
3	3.32% (1.44%)
4 or more	6.25% (2.53%)
Brothers	
0	3.90% (1.23%)
1	3.84% (1.35%)
2	3.16% (1.48%)
3	1.28% (0.82%)
4 or more	4.78% (2.01%)

TABLE B3. (From figure 4.2c.) Bivariate relationship between the receipt of any formal help and more social network characteristics for individuals who report difficulty performing at least one ADL or IADL—late-middle-aged adults.

	% (*SE*) With Any Formal Help
Has Any	
Adult Daughters	
No	4.05% (1.32%)
Yes	3.38% (0.82%)
Adult Sons	
No	2.22% (0.88%)
Yes	4.17% (0.76%)
Sisters	
No	1.41% (0.54%)
Yes	4.48% (0.80%)
Brothers	
No	3.90% (1.23%)
Yes	3.57% (0.68%)
Living Parents	
No	3.45% (0.76%)
Yes	3.71% (0.98%)

TABLE B4. (From figure 4.3a.) Bivariate relationship between the receipt of any formal help and select sociodemographic characteristics for individuals who report difficulty performing at least one ADL or IADL—young old adults.

	% (*SE*) With Any Formal Help		% (*SE*) With Any Formal Help
Gender		**Insurance**	
Male	9.34% (1.37%)	*Medicare (1/0)*	
Female	4.11% (0.89%)	No	6.07% (3.26%)
		Yes	7.31% (0.89%)
Marital Status			
Married/partnered	4.92% (1.16%)	*Medicaid (1/0)*	
Divorced/separated	12.80% (3.9%)	No	4.48% (0.69%)
Widowed	8.99% (2.08%)	Yes	18.67% (3.34%)
Never married	10.41% (4.02%)		
		Private (1/0)	
Race/Ethnicity		No	8.44% (1.25%)
Non-Hispanic White	6.14% (0.93%)	Yes	4.47% (1.31%)
Non-Hispanic Black	6.61% (2.57%)		
Hispanic	17.50% (2.78%)	*Uninsured (1/0)*	
Other	2.64% (2.68%)	No	7.27% (0.89%)
		Yes	6.03% (5.94%)
Education			
Less than high school	8.21% (1.49%)	**Household Income**	
High school	7.37% (1.69%)		
More than high school	5.62% (1.59%)	Quintile 1	11.31% (1.92%)
		Quintile 2	6.96% (1.61%)
Currently Working		Quintile 3	3.22% (1.45%)
No	7.96% (0.99%)	Quintile 4	1.82% (1.09%)
Yes	0.63% (0.64%)	Quintile 5	6.06% (3.04%)

TABLE B5. (From figure 4.3b.) Bivariate relationship between the receipt of any formal help and select social network characteristics for individuals who report difficulty performing at least one ADL or IADL—young old adults.

	% (*SE*) With Any Formal Help
Number of	
Daughters	
0	11.09% (2.30%)
1	5.59% (1.32%)
2	8.50% (1.92%)
3	4.06% (1.53%)
4 or more	4.25% (2.39%)
Sons	
0	10.02% (1.90%)
1	8.49% (1.7%)
2	4.24% (1.45%)
3	7.27% (2.39%)
4 or more	4.40% (2.01%)
Sisters	
0	7.49% (1.58%)
1	5.33% (1.65%)
2	11.18% (2.49%)
3	6.10% (2.86%)
4 or more	6.31% (2.85%)
Brothers	
0	10.85% (1.74%)
1	5.96% (1.37%)
2	2.69% (1.24%)
3	4.91% (1.83%)
4 or more	7.93% (3.87%)

TABLE B6. (From figure 4.3c.) Bivariate relationship between the receipt of any formal help and more social network characteristics for individuals who report difficulty performing at least one ADL or IADL—young old adults.

	% (*SE*) With Any Formal Help
Has Any	
Adult Daughters	
No	11.09% (2.30%)
Yes	5.94% (0.81%)
Adult Sons	
No	10.02% (1.90%)
Yes	6.42% (0.90%)
Sisters	
No	7.49% (1.58%)
Yes	7.22% (1.11%)
Brothers	
No	10.85% (1.74%)
Yes	5.12% (1.04%)
Living Parents	
No	8.16% (1.06%)
Yes	2.58% (1.33%)
Anyone in Network	
No	14.64% (9.96%)
Yes	7.16% (0.90%)

Table B7. (From figure 4.4a.) Bivariate relationship between the receipt of any formal help and select sociodemographic characteristics for individuals who report difficulty performing at least one ADL or IADL—older old adults.

	% (*SE*) With Any Formal Help		% (*SE*) With Any Formal Help
Gender		**Insurance**	
Male	17.39% (1.38%)	*Medicare (1/0)*	
Female	9.90% (1.80%)	No	10.31% (4.13%)
		Yes	14.93% (1.30%)
Marital Status			
Married/ partnered	6.78% (1.45%)	*Medicaid (1/0)*	
Divorced/ separated	16.85% (4.62%)	No	12.07% (1.00%)
		Yes	31.58% (3.64%)
Widowed	20.24% (1.75%)		
Never married	21.89% (4.52%)		
		Private (1/0)	
Race/Ethnicity		No	16.33% (1.71%)
		Yes	10.68% (1.61%)
Non-Hispanic White	13.95% (1.24%)		
Non-Hispanic Black	16.11% (3.43%)	*Uninsured (1/0)*	
Hispanic	24.65% (2.74%)	No	14.88% (1.30%)
Other	19.26% (6.98%)	Yes	0% (0%)
Education		**Household Income**	
Less than high school	15.91% (1.95%)		
High school	14.69% (1.46%)	Quintile 1	20.05% (2.27%)
More than high school	13.07% (1.85%)	Quintile 2	13.32% (1.77%)
		Quintile 3	8.7% (1.97%)
Currently Working		Quintile 4	9.49% (2.64%)
No	15.19% (1.32%)	Quintile 5	12.34% (3.65%)
Yes	3.44% (3.34%)		

TABLE B8. (From figure 4.4b.) Bivariate relationship between the receipt of any formal help and select social network characteristics for individuals who report difficulty performing at least one ADL or IADL—older old adults.

	% (*SE*) With Any Formal Help
Number of	
Daughters	
0	16.89% (1.72%)
1	14.24% (1.42%)
2	12.47% (2.51%)
3	19.92% (3.67%)
4 or more	10.01% (3.60%)
Sons	
0	16.05% (1.78%)
1	14.67% (1.76%)
2	12.33% (2.28%)
3	16.91% (3.77%)
4 or more	13.93% (4.76%)
Sisters	
0	16.44% (1.46%)
1	13.29% (1.84%)
2	13.37% (2.44%)
3	11.90% (3.66%)
4 or more	10.96% (3.50%)
Brothers	
0	16.19% (1.33%)
1	13.04% (2.29%)
2	11.95% (2.94%)
3	6.97% (2.76%)
4 or more	22.93% (8.19%)

TABLE B9. (From figure 4.4c.) Bivariate relationship between the receipt of any formal help and more social network characteristics for individuals who report difficulty performing at least one ADL or IADL—older old adults.

	% (*SE*) With Any Formal Help
Has Any	
Adult Daughters	
No	16.89% (1.72%)
Yes	14.01% (1.43%)
Adult Sons	
No	16.05% (1.78%)
Yes	14.24% (1.44%)
Sisters	
No	16.44% (1.46%)
Yes	12.93% (1.58%)
Brothers	
No	16.19% (1.33%)
Yes	12.63% (1.9%)
Anyone in Network	
No	31.29% (6.05%)
Yes	14.25% (1.32%)

Appendix C

Multivariate Results of Total Hours of Care

Table C1. OLS regression of logged hours of total care in the past month.

	β (*SE*)
Constant	–0.49 (0.2)***
Age (ref: 75+)	
50–64	–0.37 (0.1)***
65–74	–0.21 (0.1)*
Number of ADL Difficulties	0.11 (0.02)***
Number of IADL Difficulties	–0.37 (0.1)***
Number of Nights in Hospital	–0.21 (0.1)**
	0.11 (0.02)
Number of Days in Bed	0.31 (0.03)*
General Health	0.01 (0)*
Wheelchair Use	–0.05 (0.08)***
Psychological Disorder	0.05 (0.02)
Cognitive Impairment	0 (0)***
Pain	0.50 (0.08)**
Number of Medical Conditions	–0.01 (0.08)
Body Mass Index (ref: 18.5 to < 40)	
Underweight (BMI < 18.5)	0.39 (0.11)
Morbidly obese (BMI > 40)	–0.24 (0.08)
Currently Working	0.02 (0.03)
Male	0.22 (0.13)***
Lives Alone	–0.02 (0.14)***
Education (ref: high school)	
Less than high school	–0.26 (0.14)
More than high school	–0.26 (0.07)

(*continued on next page*)

Table C1. *(continued)*

	β (*SE*)
Race/Ethnicity (ref: non-Hispanic White)	
Non-Hispanic Black	–0.75 (0.1)
Hispanic	–0.06 (0.08)
Other	–0.01 (0.09)
Household Income (ref: lowest quintile)	
Quintile 2	–0.02 (0.1)
Quintile 3	0.04 (0.24)
Quintile 4	0.24 (0.16)
Quintile 5	0.15 (0.11)
Number of Informal Caregivers	0.08 (0.11)***
Primary Caregiver (ref: spouse)	
Child	–0.02 (0.13)**
Other relative	–0.13 (0.14)**
Nonrelative	0.28 (0.03)*
Formal	–0.28 (0.09)
Receives Any Formal Assistance	–0.39 (0.13)***
***N*, R^2**	2,156, .37
***F*(*nDF*, *dDF*)**	(33, 20) = 41.95
prob. > *F*	0.000

*$p < .05$. **$p < .01$. ***$p < .001$.

TABLE C2. OLS regression of logged hours of total care with age interactions.

	Model 1 β (*SE*)	Model 2 β (*SE*)
Constant	3.13 (0.17)***	3.23 (0.19)***
Age (ref: 75+)		
50–64	–0.26 (0.12)*	–0.42 (0.1)***
65–74	0.01 (0.13)	–0.20 (0.1)*
Primary Caregiver (ref: spouse)		
Child	–0.11 (0.10)	
Other relative	–0.08 (0.19)	
Nonrelative	–0.49 (0.23)*	
Formal	–0.06 (0.18)	
Receives Any Formal Assistance		0.54 (0.11)***
Age × Primary Caregiver Interaction (ref: older old, spouse)		
50–64 × Child	–0.28 (0.16)	
50–64 × Other relative	–0.54 (0.27)*	
50–64 × Nonrelative	0.23 (0.50)	
50–64 × Formal	0.29 (0.28)	
65–74 × Child	–0.33 (0.17)	
65–74 × Other relative	–0.58 (0.37)	
65–74 × Nonrelative	–0.49 (0.64)	
65–74 × Formal	–0.49 (0.25)*	
Age × Formal Care Interaction (ref: older old, no formal care)		
50–64 × Formal care		0.53 (0.21)*
65–74 × Formal care		–0.09 (0.18)
***N*, R^2**	2,156, .37	2,156, 0.37
***F*(*nDF*, *dDF*)**	(41, 12) = 41.12	(35, 18) = 41.95
prob. > *F*	0.000	0.000

*$p < .05$. **$p < .01$. ***$p < .001$.

References

Administration on Aging (AoA). (n.d.). *Services for seniors*. Retrieved January 15, 2004, from Administration on Aging Web site: http://www.aoa.gov/eldfam/Service_Options/Service_Options.asp

Agree, E. M., & Freedman, V. A. (2003). A comparison of assistive technology and personal care in alleviating disability and unmet need. *Gerontologist, 43*, 335–344.

Ajrouch, K. J., Antonucci, T. C., & Janevic, M. R. (2001). Social networks among blacks and whites: The interaction between race and age. *Journal of Gerontology: Social Sciences, 56B*, S112–S118.

Allen, K. R., Blieszner, R., & Roberto, K. A. (2000). Families in the middle and later years: A review and critique of research in the 1990s. *Journal of Marriage and the Family, 62*, 911–926.

Allen, S. M. (1994). Gender differences in spousal caregiving and unmet need for care. *Journal of Gerontology: Social Sciences, 49*, S187–S195.

Allen, S. M., & Ciambrone, D. (2003). Community care for people with disability: Blurring boundaries between formal and informal caregivers. *Qualitative Health Research, 13*, 207–226.

Allen, S. M., Foster, A., & Berg, K. (2001). Receiving help at home: The interplay of human and technological assistance. *Journal of Gerontology: Social Sciences, 56B*, S374–S382.

Allen, S. M., Goldscheider, F., & Ciambrone, D. A. (1999). Gender roles, martial intimacy, and nomination of spouse as primary caregiver. *The Gerontologist, 39*, 150–158.

Allen, S. M., & Mor, V. (1997). The prevalence and consequences of unmet need: Contrasts between older and younger adults with disability. *Medical Care, 35*, 1132–1148.

Angermeyer, M. C., Beck, M., Dietrich, S., & Holzinger, A. (2001). The stigma of mental illness: Patients' anticipations and experiences. *Psychiatric Services, 52*, 1627–1632.

Baltes, P. B. (1987). Theoretical propositions of life-span developmental psychology: On the dynamics between growth and decline. *Developmental Pscychology, 23*, 611–626.

Brown, M. E., Bindman, A. B., & Lurie, N. (1998). Monitoring the consequences of uninsurance: A review of methodologies. *Medical Care Research and Review, 55*, 177–210.

Bruce, B., Fries, J. (2003). The Stanford Health Assessment Questionnaire: A review of its history, issues, progress, and documentation. *Journal of Rheumatology, 30*, 167–178.

Cantor, M. H., Brennan, M., & Sainz, A. (1994). The importance of ethnicity in the social support systems of older New Yorkers: A longitudinal perspective (1970–1990). *Journal of Gerontological Social Work, 22*, 95–128.

Centers for Disease Control and Prevention (CDC). (2001). Prevalence of disabilities and associated health conditions among adults—United States, 1999. *Morbidity and Mortality Weekly Report, 50*, 120–125.

Centers for Disease Control and Prevention (CDC). (2002). State-specific prevalence of obesity among adults with disabilities—Eight States and the District of Columbia, 1998–1999. *Morbidity and Mortality Weekly Report, 51*, 805–810.

Centers for Medicare and Medicaid Services. (n.d.). *Medicare eligibility criteria*. Retrieved January 15, 2004, from Centers for Medicare and Medicaid Services Web site: http://www.medicare.gov/MedicareEligibility/Home.asp?dest=NAV|Home|GeneralEnrollment#TabTop

Collins, K. S., Schoen, C., Joseph, S., et al. (1999). *Informal caregiving*. The Commonwealth Fund. Retrieved April 23, 2008 from The Commonwealth Fund Web site: http://www.commonwealthfund.org/usr_doc/caregiving_fact_sheet.pdf?section=4039

Congressional Budget Office. (2004, April). *Financing long-term care for the elderly*. Retrieved February 10, 2006, from Congressional Budget Office Web site: http://www.cbo.gov/ftpdocs/54xx/doc5400/04-26-LongTermCare.pdf

Crimmins, E., & Ingegneri, D. (1990). Interaction and living arrangements of older parents and their children: Past trends, present determinants, future implications. *Research on Aging, 12*, 3–35.

DeJong, G., & Brannont, R. (1998). Trends in services directed to working-age people with physical disabilities. In S. Allen & V. Mor (Eds.), *Living in the community with disability: Service needs, use, and systems* (pp. 168–196). New York: Springer.

Desai, M. M., Lentzner, H., & Weeks, J. D. (2001). Unmet need for personal assistance with activities of daily living among older adults. *Gerontologist, 41*, 82–88.

Diehr, P., Patrick, D., Hedrick, S., Rothman, M., Grembowski, D., Raghunathan, T. E., et al. (1995). Including deaths when measuring health status over time. *Medical Care, 33*(Suppl. 4), AS164–AS172.

Diehr, P., Williamson, J., Burke, G., & Psaty, B. (2002). The aging and dying processes and the health of older adults. *Journal of Clinical Epidemiology, 55*, 269–278.

Dilworth-Anderson, P., Williams, I. C., & Gibson, B. E. (2002). Issues of race, ethnicity, and culture in caregiving research: A 20-year review (1980–2000). *The Gerontologist, 42*, 237–272.

Doty, P., Jackson, M. E., & Crown, W. (1998). The impact of female caregivers' employment status on patterns of formal and informal eldercare. *The Gerontologist, 38*, 331–341.

Downs, B. (2003). Current population reports (P20–548). In *Fertility of American women: June 2002*. Washington, DC: U.S. Census Bureau. Retrieved April 23, 2008 from U.S. Census Bureau Web site: http://www.census.biz/prod/2003pubs/p20-548.pdf

Elashoff, J. D. (2002). *NQuery Advisor, Version 5.0. user's guide*. Los Angeles: Statistical Solutions, Ltd.

Elder, G. H., Jr. (1975). Age differentiation and the life course. *Annual Review of Sociology, 1*, 165–190.

Elder, G. H., Jr. (1978). Family history and the life course. In T. K. Hareven (Ed.), *Transitions* (pp. 17–64). New York: Academic Press.

Elder, G. H., Jr. (1994). Time, human agency, and social change: Perspectives on the life course. *Social Psychology Quarterly, 57*, 4–15.

Elder, G. H., Jr., & Johnson, M. K. (2002). The life course and aging: Challenges, lessons, and new directions. In R. A. Settersten, Jr. (Ed.), *Invitation to the life course: Toward new understandings of later life* (pp. 49–81). Amityville, NY: Baywood.

Faber, A., & Wasserman, S. (2001). Social support and social networks: Synthesis and review. In J. Levy & B. Pescosolido (Eds.), *Advances in medical sociology, Volume 8: Social networks and health* (pp. 29–72). Stamford, CT: JAI Press.

Freedman, V. A., Martin, L. G., & Schoeni, R. F. (2002). Recent trends in disability and functioning among older adults in the United States: A systematic review. *Journal of the American Medical Association, 288*, 3137–3146.

Gaugler, J. E., Kane, R. L., Kane, R. A., & Newcomer, R. (2005). Unmet care needs and key outcomes in dementia. *Journal of the American Geriatrics Society, 53*, 2098–2105.

George, L. (2002). What life-course perspectives offer the study of aging and health. In R. A. Settersten, Jr. (Ed.), *Invitation to the life course: Toward new understandings of later life* (pp. 161–188). Amityville, NY: Baywood.

Gitlin, L. (2003). Conducting research on home environments: Lessons learned and new directions. *The Gerontologist, 43*, 628–637.

Glasgow, N. (2000). Rural/urban patterns of aging and caregiving in the United States. *Journal of Family Issues, 21*, 611–631.

Goldscheider, F. (1990). The aging of the gender revolution: What do we know and what do we need to know? *Research on Aging, 12*, 531–545.

Harrison, B., & Bluestone, B. (1998). The crisis of the American dream. In T. Shapiro (Ed.), *Great divides* (pp. 179–191). Mountain View, CA: Mayfield.

Health and Retirement Study. (2000). *Core public use dataset.* Produced and distributed by the University of Michigan with funding from the National Institute on Aging (Grant No. NIA U01AG009740). Ann Arbor: University of Michigan.

Ho, A., Collins, S. R., Davis, K., & Doty, M. M. (2005). *A look at working-age caregivers' roles, health concerns, and need for support*. The Commonwealth Fund. Retrieved April 23, 2008, from The Commonwealth Fund Web site: http://www.commonwealthfund.org/usr_doc/854_Ho_lookatworking caregiversroles_IB.pdf?section=4039

Hobbs, F., & Stoops, N. (2002). *Demographic trends in the 20th century* (Census 2000 Special Report No. CENSR-4). Washington, DC: U.S. Census Bureau. Retrieved September 11, 2003, from U.S. Census Bureau Web site: http://www.census.gov/prod/2002pubs/censr-4.pdf

Hogan, D., Eggebeen, D., & Clogg, C. (1993). The structure of intergenerational exchanges in American families. *American Journal of Sociology, 98*, 1428–1458.

Holtz-Eakin, D. (2005, April 27). *CBO testimony of the cost and financing of long-term care services before the Subcommittee on Health Committee on Energy and Commerce, U.S. House of Representatives*. Retrieved February 10, 2006, from Congressional Budget Office Web site: http://www.cbo.gov/ftpdocs/63xx/doc6316/04-27-LongTermCare_testimony.pdf

Horowitz, A. (1985). Reciprocity and affection: Past influences on current caregiving. *Journal of Gerontological Social Work, 5*, 5–20.

Iezzoni, L. (2003). *When walking fails*. Berkeley: University of California Press.

Jette, A., Tennstedt, S., & Branch, L. (1992). Stability of informal long-term care. *Journal of Aging and Health, 4*, 193–211.

Johnson, C. (2000). Perspectives on American kinship in the later 1990s. *Journal of Marriage and the Family, 62*, 623–639.

Johnson, R. W., Moon, M., & Davidoff, A. J. (2002). *A Medicare buy-in for the near elderly: Design issues and potential effects on coverage*. Menlo Park, CA: Henry J. Kaiser Family Foundation.

Kalton, G., & Kasprzyk, D. (1986). The treatment of missing survey data. *Statistics Canada, 12*, 1–16.

Karner, T. (2001). Caring for an aging society: Cohort values and eldercare services. *Journal of Aging and Social Policy, 13*, 15–36.

Katz, S., & Akpom, A. (1976). A measure of primary sociobiological functions. *International Journal of Health Services, 6*, 493–508.

Katz, S. J., Kabeto, M., & Langa, K. M. (2000). Gender disparities in the receipt of home care for elderly people with disability in the United States. *Journal of the American Medical Association, 284*, 3022–3027.

Kemper, P. (1988). The evaluation of the national long term care demonstration: Overview of the findings. *Health Services Research, 23*, 161–174.

Kertzer, D. I., & Keith, J. (Eds.). (1984). *Age and anthropological theory*. Ithaca, NY: Cornell University Press.

Klein, B. E., Klein, R., Knudston, M. D., & Lee, K. E. (2005). Frailty, morbidity, and survival. *Archives of Gerontology and Geriatrics, 41*, 141–149.

Komisar, H. L., Feder, J., & Kasper, J. D. (2005). Unmet long-term care needs: An analysis of Medicare-Medicaid dual eligibles. *Inquiry, 42*, 171–182.

Kramarow, E. (1995). The elderly who live alone in the United States: Historical perspectives on household change. *Demography, 32*, 335–352.

Kreider, R., & Simmons, T. (October 2003). *Marital status: 2000 census 2000 brief.* Washington, DC: U.S. Department of Commerce Economics and Statistics Administration. Retrieved April 23, 2008, from U.S. Census Bureau Web site: www.census.gov/prod/2003pubs/c2kbr-30.pdf

LaPlante, M. (1993). *Disability, health insurance coverage, and utilization of acute health services in the United States* (Disability Statistics Report No. 4). Washington, DC: National Institute on Disability and Rehabilitation Research, U.S. Department of Health and Human Services.

LaPlante, M., Harrington, C., & Kang, T. (2002). Estimating paid and unpaid hours of personal assistance services in activities of daily living provided to adults living at home. *Health Services Research, 37*, 397–415.

LaPlante, M., Kaye, H. S., Kang, T., & Harrington, C. (2004). Unmet need for personal assistance services: Estimating the shortfall in hours of help and adverse consequences. *Journal of Gerontology, 59B*, S98–S108.

Lawton, M. P. (1971). The functional assessment of elderly people. *Journal of the American Geriatrics Society, 19*, 465.

Levy, F. (1998). *The new dollars and dreams*. New York: Russell Sage Foundation.

Lima, J. C., & Allen, S. M. (2001). Targeting risk for unmet need: Not enough help versus no help at all. *Journal of Gerontology, 56B*, S302–S310.

Lima, J., Allen, S., Goldscheider, F., & Intrator, O. (2008). Spousal caregiving in late midlife versus older ages: Implications of work and family obligations. *Journal of Gerontology: Social Sciences, 63B*, S229–S238.

Lindsay, J., & Anderson, L. (2004). Dementia/Alzheimer's disease. *BMC Women's Health, 4*(Suppl. 1), S20.

Link, B. G., Phelan J. C., Bresnahan, M., Stueve, A., & Pescosolido, B. A. (2004). Public conceptions of mental illness: Labels, causes, dangerousness, and social distance. *International Journal of Social Psychiatry, 50*, 153–162.

Litwak, E. (1985). *Helping the elderly: The complementary roles of informal networks and formal systems*. New York: Guilford Press.

Long, S. K., King, J., & Coughlin, T. A. (2005–2006). The implications of unmet need for future health care use: Findings for a sample of disabled Medicaid beneficiaries in New York. *Inquiry, 42*, 413–420.

Macunovich, D. J., Easterlin, R. A., Schaeffer, C. M., & Crimmons, E. M. (1995). Echoes of the baby boom and bust: Recent and prospective changes in living alone among elderly widows in the United States. *Demography, 32*, 17–28.

McCarty, D., & Levine, H. (1999). Needs of people with chronic and disabling conditions. In M. Lillie-Blanton, R. Martinez, B. Lyons, & D. Rowland (Eds.), *Access to health care: Promises and prospects for low-income Americans* (Chapter 4, pp. 61–72). Washington, DC: The Kaiser Commission on Medicaid and the Uninsured.

McTigue, K., Larson, J. C., Valoski, A., Burke, G., Kotchen, J., Lewis, C. E., et al. (2006). Mortality and cardiac and vascular outcomes in extremely obese women. *Journal of the American Medical Association, 296*, 79–86.

McWilliams, J. M., Zaslavsky, A. M., Meara, E., & Ayanian, J. Z. (2003). Impact of Medicare coverage on basic clinical services for previously uninsured adults. *Journal of the American Medical Association, 290*, 757–764.

Messeri, P., Silverstein, M., & Litwak, E. (1993). Choosing optimal support groups: A review and reformulation. *Journal of Health and Social Behavior, 24*, 122–137.

Miller, N. A. (2005). State strategies to support community-based long term care for the elderly. *Journal of Health and Social Policy, 20*(4), 1–30.

Moen, P., Robison, J., & Fields, V. (1994). Women's work and caregiving roles: A life course approach. *Journal of Gerontology, 49*, S176–S186.

Moon, M. (1996). *Medicare now and in the future* (2nd ed.). Washington, DC: The Urban Institute Press.

Moon, M. (2005). Sustaining Medicare as an age-related program. In R. B. Hudson (Ed.), *The new politics of old age policy* (pp. 205–218). Baltimore: Johns Hopkins University Press.

Mor, V., Allen, S. M., Siegel, K., & Houts, P. (1992). Determinants of need and unmet need among cancer patients residing at home. *Health Services Research, 27*, 337–360.

National Institute on Aging (NIA). (1999, March). The declining disability of older Americans. *Research Highlight in the Demography and Economics of Aging, 5.*

Neal, M. B., Ingersoll-Dayton, B., & Starrels, M. E. (1997). Gender and relationship differences in caregiving patterns and consequences among employed caregivers. *The Gerontologist, 37*, 804–816.

O'Rand, A. M. (2005). When old age begins: Implications for health, work, and retirement. In R. B. Hudson (Ed.), *The new politics of old age policy* (pp. 109–128). Baltimore: Johns Hopkins University Press.

Ory, M. G., Hoffman, R. R., III, Yee, J. L., Tennstedt, S., & Schulz, R. (1999). Prevalence and impact of caregiving: A detailed comparison between dementia and nondementia caregivers. *Gerontologist, 39*, 177–185.

Pastor, P. N., Makuc, D. M., Reuben, C. M., & Xia, H. (2002). *Health, United States, 2002, with chartbook on trends in the health of Americans*. Hyattsville, MD: National Center for Health Statistics. Retrieved June 12, 2006, from Centers for Disease Control Web site: http://www.cdc.gov/nchs/data/hus/hus02.pdf

Paul, C., Mason, W. M., McCaffrey, D., & Fox, S. A. (2003, October 1). *What should we do about missing data? (A case study using logistic regression with missing data on a single covariate)* (On-Line Working Paper Series No. CCPR-028-03). Los Angeles: University of California, California Center for Population Research.

Penning, M. J. (2002). Hydra revisited: Substituting formal for self—and informal in-home care among older adults with disabilities. *The Gerontologist, 42*, 4–16.

Pezzin, L. E., &. Schone, B. S. (1999). Parental marital disruption and intergenerational transfers: An analysis of lone elderly parents and their children. *Demography, 36*, 287–297.

Phelan, J. C., Bromet, E., & Link, B. (1998). Psychiatric illness and family stigma. *Schizophrenia Bulletin, 24*, 115–126.

Pol, L., Mueller, K., & Adidam, P. (2000). Health insurance in the near elderly population. *Population Research and Policy Review, 19*, 97–112.

Quadagno, J. (2005). *One nation uninsured: Why the U.S. has no national health insurance*. New York: Oxford University Press.

Resnik, L., Lapane, K. L., &. Allen, S. M. (2005). Obesity and receipt of personal care assistance for people with mobility impairments. *Obesity Research, 13*, 1307–1310.

Riley, M. W., Johnson, M. E., & Foner, A. (Eds.). (1972). *Aging and society, Vol. 3: A sociology of age stratification*. New York: Russell Sage.

Roschelle, A. R. (1997). *No more kin: Exploring race, class, and gender in family networks*. Thousand Oaks, CA: Sage.

Rubin, D. B. (1996). Multiple imputation after 18+ years. *Journal of the American Statistics Association, 91*, 473–489.

Ruggles, S. (1995). Living arrangements of the elderly in America, 1880–1980. In T. Hareven (Ed.), *Aging and generational relations over the life course: Historical and cross-cultural perspectives* (pp. 254–271). New York: W. de Gruyter.

Sands, L. P., Wang, Y., McCabe, G. P., Jennings, K., Eng, C., & Covinsky, K. E. (2006). Rates of acute care admissions for frail older people living with met versus unmet activity of daily living needs. *Journal of the American Geriatrics Society, 54*, 339–344.

Schoen, C., Simantov, E., Duchon, L., & Davis, K. (2000). *Counting on Medicare: Perspectives and concerns of Americans ages 50 to 70*. New York: Commonwealth Fund.

Settersten, R. A., Jr. (2002). Rethinking social policy: Lessons of a life-course perspective. In R. A. Settersten, Jr. (Ed.), *Invitation to the life course: Toward new understandings of later life* (pp. 191–221). Amityville, NY: Baywood.

Shea, D. G., Short, P. F., & Powell, M. P. (2001). Betwixt and between: Targeting coverage reforms to those approaching Medicare. *Health Affairs (Millwood), 20*, 219–230.

Shirk, C. (2007, May 30). *Trading places: Real choice system change grants and the reform movement to community-based long term care supports* (Issue Brief No. 822). Washington, DC: National Health Policy Forum.

Silverstein, M. (1995). Stability and change in temporal distance between the elderly and their children. *Demography, 32*, 29–45.

Silverstein, M., Conroy, S. J., Wang, H., Giarrusso, R., & Bengtson, V. L. (2002). Reciprocity in parent-child relations over the adult life course. *Journal of Gerontology, 57B*, S8–S13.

Soldo, B., & Hill, M. S. (1995). Family structure and transfer measures in the HRS: Background and overview. *Journal of Human Resources, 30*(Suppl. 1995), S108–S117.

Speare, A., & Avery, R. (1993). Who helps whom in older parent-child families? *Journal of Gerontology, 48*, S64–S73.

Statacorp. (2003). *Stata statistical software: Release 8.0*. College Station, TX: Stata Corporation.

Steinmetz, E. (2006). Current population reports (P70–107). In *American with Disabilities: 2002*. Washington, DC: U.S. Census Bureau. Retrieved June 8, 2006, from U.S. Census Bureau Web site: http://www.census.gov/prod/2006pubs/p70-107.pdf

Stewart, P. (2007). Who is kin? Family definition and African American families. *Journal of Human Behavior in the Social Environment, 15*, 163–181.

Stoller, E. P. (1990). Males as helpers: The role of sons, relatives, and friends. *The Gerontologist, 30*, 228–235.

Stommel, M., Given, C., & Given, B. (1998). Racial differences in the division of labor between primary and secondary caregivers. *Research on Aging, 20*, 199–217.

Stone, R., Cafferata, G., & Sangl, J. (1987). Caregivers of the frail elderly: A national profile. *The Gerontologist, 27*, 616–626.

Tennstedt, S., Harrow, B., & Crawford, S. (1996). Informal care vs. formal services: Changes in patterns of care over time. *Journal of Aging and Social Policy, 7*(3/4), 71–91.

Turner, H. (1996). Determinants of perceived family support and conflict: Life course variations among the physically disabled. *International Journal of Aging and Human Development, 42*, 21–41.

U.S. Census Bureau. (2007). *Current population survey, 2006 annual social and economic supplement table A1. Marital status of people 15 years and over, by age, sex, personal earnings, race, and Hispanic origin.* Washington, DC: Author. Retrieved July 6, 2007, from www.census.gov/population/socdemo/hh-fam/cps2006/tabA10all.xls

U.S. Census Bureau, Public Information Office. (2001, June 1). *Census Bureau facts for feature: Older American month celebrated in May* (CB01-FF.07). Washington, DC: Author. Retrieved January 15, 2004, from U.S. Census Bureau Web site: http://www.census.gov/Press-Release/www/2001/cb01ff07.html

van den Berg, B., & Spauwen, P. (2006). Measurement of informal care: An empirical study into the valid measurement of time spent on informal caregiving. *Health Economics, 15*, 447–460.

Wallace, R., & Herzog, A. (1995). Overview of the health measures in the Health and Retirement Study. *The Journal of Human Resources, 30*(Suppl.), S84–S107.

Wallace, S. P., Levy-Storms, L., Kington, R. S., & Andersen, R. M. (1998). The persistence of race and ethnicity in the use of long-term care. *Journal of Gerontology, 53B*, S104–S112.

Wang, Q. (2005, July). *Disability and American families: 2000* (Census 2000 Special Report No. CENSR-23). Washington, DC: U.S. Census Bureau. Retrieved April 23, 2008, from U.S. Census Bureau Web site: http://www.census.gov/prod/2005pubs/censr-23.pdf

Weissman, J. S., & Epstein, A. M. (1994). *Falling through the safety net: Insurance status and access to health care*. Baltimore: The Johns Hopkins University Press.

Williams, C. (2004, September). The sandwich generation [Electronic version]. *Perspectives on Labour and Income—Statistics Canada, 5*(9), 5–12.

Wolff, J. L., & Kasper, J. D. (2006). Caregivers of frail elders: Updating a national profile. *Gerontologist, 46*, 344–356.

World Health Organization (WHO). (2001). *International classification of functioning, disability, and health: ICF*. Geneva, Switzerland: Author. Retrieved April 23, 2008, from WHO Web site: http://www.who.int/classifications/icf/en/

Index

Made in the USA
Monee, IL
12 November 2026

f94a0e76-4554-4654-a782-756f7c11d82dR01